Foot and Ankle Arthroscopy

Guest Editor

LAURENCE G. RUBIN, DPM, FACFAS

CLINICS IN PODIATRIC MEDICINE AND SURGERY

www.podiatric.theclinics.com

Consulting Editor

THOMAS ZGONIS, DPM, FACFAS

July 2011 • Volume 28 • Number 3

SAUNDERS an imprint of ELSEVIER, Inc.

W.B. SAUNDERS COMPANY
A Division of Elsevier Inc.

1600 John F. Kennedy Boulevard ● Suite 1800 ● Philadelphia, Pennsylvania 19103-2899

http://www.theclinics.com

CLINICS IN PODIATRIC MEDICINE AND SURGERY Volume 28, Number 3
July 2011 ISSN 0891-8422, ISBN-13: 978-1-4557-1050-8

Editor: Patrick Manley

Clinics in Podiatric Medicine and Surgery (ISSN 0891-8422) is published quarterly by Elsevier Inc., 360 Park Avenue South, New York, NY 10010-1710. Months of issue are January, April, July, and October. Business and Editorial Offices: 1600 John F. Kennedy Blvd., Ste. 1800, Philadelphia, PA 19103-2899. Customer Service Office: 3251 Riverport Lane, Maryland Heights, MO 63043. Periodicals postage paid at New York, NY and additional mailing offices. Subscription prices are $270.00 per year for US individuals, $385.00 per year for US institutions, $137.00 per year for US students and residents, $324.00 per year for Canadian individuals, $477.00 for Canadian institutions, $384.00 for international individuals, $477.00 per year for international institutions and $193.00 per year for Canadian and foreign students/residents. To receive student/resident rate, orders must be accompanied by name of affiliated institution, date of term, and the *signature* of program/residency coordinator on institution letterhead. Orders will be billed at individual rate until proof of status is received. Foreign air speed delivery is included in all *Clinics* subscription prices. All prices are subject to change without notice. POSTMASTER: Send address changes to *Clinics in Podiatric Medicine and Surgery*, Elsevier Health Sciences Division, Subscription Customer Service, 3251 Riverport Lane, Maryland Heights, MO 63043. **Customer Service: 1-800-654-2452 (US). From outside of the US, call 314-447-8871. Fax: 314-447-8029. E-mail: JournalsCustomerService-usa@elsevier.com (for print support); JournalsOnlineSupport-usa@elsevier.com (for online support).**

Reprints. For copies of 100 or more of articles in this publication, please contact the Commercial Reprints Department, Elsevier Inc., 360 Park Avenue South, New York, NY 10010-1710. Tel.: 212-633-3812; Fax: 212-462-1935; E-mail: reprints@elsevier.com.

Clinics in Podiatric Medicine and Surgery is covered in *MEDLINE/PubMed (Index Medicus)* and *EMBASE/Excerpta Medica.*

Printed and bound by CPI Group (UK) Ltd, Croydon, CR0 4YY
Transferred to Digital Print 2012

CLINICS IN PODIATRIC MEDICINE AND SURGERY

CONSULTING EDITOR
THOMAS ZGONIS, DPM, FACFAS

Contributors

CONSULTING EDITOR

THOMAS ZGONIS, DPM, FACFAS
Director, Podiatric Surgical Residency and Reconstructive Fellowship Programs; Chief, Division of Podiatric Medicine and Surgery; Associate Professor, Department of Orthopedic Surgery, The University of Texas Health Science Center at San Antonio, San Antonio, Texas

GUEST EDITOR

LAURENCE G. RUBIN, DPM, FACFAS
Private Practice, Richmond, Virginia

AUTHORS

SAMANTHA E. BARK, DPM
Fellow, Department of Podiatry, Palo Alto Medical Foundation, Mountain View, California

JEFFREY C. CHRISTENSEN, DPM, FACFAS
Research Director, International Foot and Ankle Foundation for Education and Research; Attending Podiatric Surgeon, Department of Orthopedics, Division of Podiatric Surgery, Swedish Medical Center, Seattle, Washington; Founder, Ankle and Foot Clinics Northwest

BENJAMIN D. CULLEN, DPM
Resident, Department of Orthopedic Surgery, Kaiser Hayward/Fremont, Fremont, California

RICHARD DERNER, DPM, FACFAS
Private Practice, Associated Foot and Ankle Centers of Northern Virginia, Lake Ridge, Virginia

LAWRENCE FORD, DPM
Director and Attending Surgeon, Kaiser San Francisco Bay Area Foot and Ankle Residency Program, Department of Orthopedics and Podiatric Surgery, Oakland, California

SPYROS GALANAKOS, MD
First Department of Orthopaedics, Athens University Medical School, ATTIKON University Hospital, Chaidari, Athens, Greece

SEAN T. GRAMBART, DPM, FACFAS
Department of Surgery, Carle Physician Group, Urbana, Illinois

GEORGE GUMANN, DPM, FACFAS
Department of Surgery, Orthopedic Clinic, Martin Army Hospital, Fort Benning, Georgia

KYLE E. HAFFNER, DPM
Chief Resident, West Houston Medical Center Podiatric Medicine and Surgery Residency Program, Houston, Texas

GRAHAM A. HAMILTON, DPM, FACFAS
Departments of Orthopedics and Podiatric Surgery, Kaiser Permanente, Antioch, California

BYRON HUTCHINSON, DPM
Director of Podiatric Medical Education, Franciscan Foot and Ankle Institute, Member, Franciscan Medical Group, Board of Directors, International Foot and Ankle Foundation, Seattle, Washington

KEITH JACOBSON, DPM, FACFAS
Private Practice, Advanced Orthopedic and Sports Medicine Specialist, Denver, Colorado

MEAGAN M. JENNINGS, DPM, FACFAS
Department of Podiatry, Palo Alto Medical Foundation, Mountain View, California

THURMOND D. LANIER, DPM, MPH
Third Year Resident, Swedish Medical Center, Seattle, Washington

MICHAEL S. LEE, DPM, FACFAS
Associate Clinical Professor, College of Podiatric Medicine and Surgery, Des Moines University, Des Moines; Foot and Ankle Surgery, Capital Orthopaedics and Sports Medicine, Clive, Iowa

ANDREAS F. MAVROGENIS, MD
First Department of Orthopaedics, Athens University Medical School, ATTIKON University Hospital, Chaidari, Athens, Greece

JASON NALDO, DPM
PGY-3, Inova Fairfax Hospital Podiatric Residency Program, Inova Fairfax Hospital, Department of Orthopaedics, Section of Podiatry, Falls Church, Virginia

ALAN NG, DPM, FACFAS
Private Practice, Advanced Orthopedic and Sports Medicine Specialist; Director/Surgical Attending, Highlands Presbyterian St Luke's Podiatric Medicine and Surgery Residency Program, Denver, Colorado

BENJAMIN D. OVERLEY Jr, DPM, FACFAS
The Sports Medicine Institute, Pottstown, Pennsylvania

PANAYIOTIS J. PAPAGELOPOULOS, MD, DSc
First Department of Orthopaedics, Athens University Medical School, ATTIKON University Hospital, Chaidari, Athens, Greece

KLEO T. PAPAPARASKEVA, MD
Department of Pathology, Athens University Medical School, ATTIKON University Hospital, Chaidari, Athens, Greece

THOMAS S. ROUKIS, DPM, PhD, FACFAS
Department of Orthopaedics, Podiatry, and Sports Medicine, Gundersen Lutheran Medical Center, La Crosse, Wisconsin

LAURENCE G. RUBIN, DPM, FACFAS
Private Practice, Richmond, Virginia

VALERIE L. SCHADE, DPM, AACFAS
Chief, Limb Preservation Service, Vascular/Endovascular Surgery Service, Department of Surgery, Madigan Healthcare System, Tacoma, Washington

TANYA J. SINGLETON, DPM
Third Year Resident, Kaiser San Francisco Bay Area Foot and Ankle Residency Program, Oakland, California

GLENN M. WEINRAUB, DPM, FACFAS
Director of Graduate Medical Education, Department of Orthopaedic Surgery, Kaiser Hayward/Fremont, Fremont, California

Contents

Foreword: Foot and Ankle Arthroscopy xiii

Thomas Zgonis

Preface: Arthroscopy of the Ankle and Foot xv

Laurence G. Rubin

Practical Aspects of Foot and Ankle Arthroscopy 441

Meagan M. Jennings and Samantha E. Bark

Arthroscopy of the foot and ankle, although sometimes technically challenging, is a useful tool for the foot and ankle surgeon. Burman in 1931 was the first to attempt arthoscopy of the ankle joint and surmised that it was not a suitable joint for arthroscopy because of its narrow intra-articular space. With the development of smaller-diameter arthroscopes and improvements in joint distraction techniques, Watanabe was the first to present a series of 28 ankle arthroscopes in 1972. At present, arthroscopy is used not only to evaluate and treat intra-articular abnormalities but also for endoscopic and tendoscopic procedures.

Preoperative Evaluation and Testing for Arthroscopy 453

Sean T. Grambart and Benjamin D. Overley Jr

Understanding when to proceed with an arthroscopy of the ankle and foot can at times be difficult. Proper preoperative planning will ensure that the correct surgical procedure is selected. Although most surgeons can determine the correct diagnosis and treatment options for the patient based on the subjective and objective examinations, advanced imaging and diagnostic injections are useful tools in difficult cases.

Soft Tissue Pathology of the Ankle 469

Benjamin D. Cullen and Glenn M. Weinraub

Derangements of the soft tissues within the ankle joint are associated with a wide variety of pathophysiology, and typically can be classified as secondary to traumatic injury, rheumatic disease, or congenital lesions. Patients often present with persistent pain, swelling, and limitations on function, usually focused on the anterior aspect of the joint. Evaluation should be guided by a detailed history and physical examination, followed by clinical, laboratory, and imaging studies as indicated. The pathophysiology, diagnosis, and management of these conditions will be the focus of this article.

Arthroscopic Treatment of Ankle Osteochondral Lesions 481

Tanya J. Singleton, Byron Hutchinson, and Lawrence Ford

Arthroscopic treatment of osteochondral lesions (OCLs) of the ankle is a popular first-line surgical option after conservative therapy has failed.

MRI is the preferred imaging modality to evaluate OCLs and aid in surgical planning. Associated soft tissue pathology must be appreciated and addressed surgically, because associated synovitis and soft tissue impingement often contribute to symptoms. The diverse treatment modalities available via arthroscopy offer simplistic and straightforward solutions for biologically and mechanically complicated pathology. Marrow-stimulating techniques, particularly microfracture, have shown good to excellent results in most patients with small (<15 mm) acute lesions, and have a low complication rate.

Arthroscopic Treatment of Anterior Ankle Impingement   491

Keith Jacobson, Alan Ng, and Kyle E. Haffner

Anterior ankle impingement is a common cause of chronic ankle pain in the athletic population. Its cause can be either soft tissue or osseous in nature. Arthroscopic debridement results in favorable and reproducible outcomes. However, in the population in which ankle instability or narrowing of the ankle joint occur, outcomes may be less favorable.

Arthroscopic Ankle Arthrodesis   511

Michael S. Lee

Arthroscopic ankle arthrodesis provides the surgeon with an alternative to traditional open techniques. Arthroscopic ankle arthrodesis has demonstrated faster union rates, decreased complications, reduced postoperative pain, and shorter hospital stays. Adherence to sound surgical techniques, particularly with regard to joint preparation, is critical for success. Although total ankle replacement continues to grow in popularity, arthroscopic ankle arthrodesis remains a viable alternative for the management of end-stage arthritic ankle.

Arthroscopically Assisted Treatment of Ankle Injuries   523

George Gumann and Graham A. Hamilton

Ankle arthroscopy is a valuable tool in the treatment of certain intra-articular fractures involving the ankle, as it provides the ability to address osteochondral injury and aids in the direct visualization for joint reduction through minimal intervention. It can sometimes be complimented by a more minimally invasive approach to fracture reduction and internal fixation. It should be noted that to perform arthroscopically assisted minimally invasive fracture approaches, the surgeon must have significant experience with traditional open techniques.

Subtalar Joint Arthroscopy   539

Laurence G. Rubin

Subtalar joint arthroscopy can be performed on a wide array of pathology. The procedure has progressed from a diagnostic test to a reconstructive procedure. Although it is not as popular as ankle arthroscopy, it is becoming more commonly discussed in the literature and is part of many arthroscopy courses. Better education along with improved instrumentation will allow more foot and ankle surgeons to treat pathology of the subtalar joint with arthroscopic techniques. This will lead to improved outcomes and lower complication rates in treating that pathology.

Small Joint Arthroscopy of the Foot   551

Richard Derner and Jason Naldo

The arthroscopic approach to small joints of the foot has made many advances in recent years, which can be directly related to the improvement of the surgical equipment. This improvement has led to more indications for the use of arthroscopy as well as minimizing the complications. Several articles recently have presented experiences in arthroscopic surgery in the small joints of the foot; however, its use is still relatively limited. Approaches to small joints of the foot involve the first metatarsophalangeal joint, tarsometatarsal joint, and Chopart joint, as well as the interphalangeal joint to the great toe and lesser toes.

Tendoscopy of the Ankle   561

Jeffrey C. Christensen and Thurmond D. Lanier

In this article, the peroneus longus and brevis, posterior tibial, Achilles, and flexor hallucis longus tendon endoscopy are discussed individually. Tendoscopic indications and surgical technique are highlighted.

Current Concepts and Techniques in Foot and Ankle Surgery

Antithrombotic Pharmacologic Prophylaxis Use During Conservative and Surgical Management of Foot and Ankle Disorders: A Systematic Review   571

Valerie L. Schade and Thomas S. Roukis

The use of antithrombotic pharmacologic prophylaxis during conservative or postoperative management of foot and ankle disorders is controversial. This article presents a systematic review of the incidence of deep venous thrombosis (DVT)/pulmonary embolus (PE) during management of foot and ankle disorders in patients who did or did not receive antithrombotic pharmacologic prophylaxis. Incidence of DVT/PE in both groups was low; however, more than half of the patients in both groups received some form of antithrombotic pharmacologic prophylaxis of varying duration, making it difficult to determine the true protective effect of antithrombotic pharmacologic prophylaxis.

Pigmented Villonodular Synovitis of the Distal Tibiofibular Joint: A Case Report   589

Andreas F. Mavrogenis, Kleo T. Papaparaskeva, Spyros Galanakos, and Panayiotis J. Papagelopoulos

Pigmented villonodular synovitis (PVNS) is a proliferative disorder of the synovium. Monoarticular involvement is the more common process. This article presents a case of PVNS with rare location at the distal tibiofibular joint and discusses the current concepts of diagnosis and treatment of this disease.

Index   599

FORTHCOMING ISSUES

October 2011
Advances in Fixation Technology for the Foot and Ankle
Patrick Burns, DPM, *Guest Editor*

January 2012
Arthrodesis of the Foot and Ankle
Steven F. Boc, DPM and
Vincent Muscarella, DPM,
Guest Editors

April 2012
Foot and Ankle Trauma
Denise Mandi, DPM, *Guest Editor*

RECENT ISSUES

April 2011
Recent Advances in Hallus Rigidus Surgery
Molly S. Judge, DPM, *Guest Editor*

January 2011
Foot and Ankle Athletic Injuries
Bob Baravarian, DPM, FACFAS,
Guest Editor

October 2010
Forefoot Pain
D. Martin Chaney, DPM, MS and
Walter W. Strash, DPM, *Guest Editors*

THE CLINICS ARE NOW AVAILABLE ONLINE!
Access your subscription at:
www.theclinics.com

Foreword

Foot and Ankle Arthroscopy

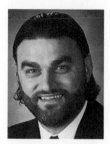

Thomas Zgonis, DPM
Consulting Editor

Arthroscopy in foot and ankle surgery has gained popularity in the last decade since the advent of new techniques, improved instrumentation, and safer means of ankle distraction. The notion of performing minimally invasive surgery utilizing arthroscopic techniques improves recovery time while decreasing the complications that are typically associated with extensile incisions and open procedures. Foot and ankle arthroscopy encompasses a broad category of indications for the treatment of both soft tissue and joint pathology. Its evolution has progressed from the initial treatment of sports-related injuries to the management of osteochondral talar defects, ankle impingement syndromes, and ankle instability. Its latest indications also include the capability of achieving an in situ ankle arthrodesis and of being used as an adjunct procedure for complex fracture repair.

The selected guest editor and invited authors have a vast experience in this field and have provided us with an excellent portrait of when to consider arthroscopy while explaining in detail novel techniques that are being tried. I congratulate the authors on their excellent work as I am confident that this edition will educate our readers in the most current surgical treatments for which foot and ankle arthroscopy can be beneficial.

Thomas Zgonis, DPM
Division of Podiatric Medicine and Surgery
Department of Orthopaedic Surgery
The University of Texas Health Science Center at San Antonio
7703 Floyd Curl Drive–MSC 7776
San Antonio, TX 78229, USA

E-mail address:
zgonis@uthscsa.edu

doi:10.1016/j.cpm.2011.06.002
0891-8422/11/$ – see front matter © 2011 Elsevier Inc. All rights reserved.
podiatric.theclinics.com

Preface

Arthroscopy of the Ankle and Foot

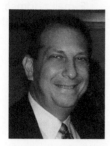

Laurence G. Rubin, DPM
Guest Editor

Arthroscopy of the ankle and foot is one of the more innovative forms of arthroscopic surgery of the human body. In its infancy, it was a more direct, but awkward diagnostic tool. It has become a mainstay in the field of foot and ankle surgery, and it continues to progress on an ongoing basis. Arthroscopic ankle fusions are becoming more commonplace and we are now able reduce fractures with less invasive techniques using arthroscopy. Similarly, arthroscopy of the foot is now becoming more established. Surgeons are routinely performing arthroscopic procedures of the subtalar and the first metatarsal phalangeal joints. The continued improvements of the medical equipment, along with the advancement in techniques and education in our profession, will lead to further development of this field of surgery.

I had the privilege of training with Harold Vogler, who coauthored the first article on ankle arthroscopy in our literature, and John Stienstra, a true pioneer in the field of ankle arthroscopy. It was their mentoring that encouraged me to develop my skills as an arthroscopist. During my tenure over the last thirteen years as a faculty member of the American College of Foot and Ankle Surgeons course in arthroscopy of the ankle and foot, I was able to share the podium with some of the most experienced and technically proficient foot and ankle surgeons in the country. It was those individuals that I asked to author articles for this edition. I would like to thank them for generously donating their time and expertise.

The authors of this *Clinics in Podiatric Medicine and Surgery* edition were asked to take the reader from the basics of equipment and technique to some of the most current procedures being performed today. Some of the authors were asked to give their incomparable experience in the more traditional pathologic conditions that foot and ankle surgeons are likely to encounter, while others were teamed up to provide a vast array of experience from multiple points of view. I hope that this edition provides

Clin Podiatr Med Surg 28 (2011) xv–xvi
doi:10.1016/j.cpm.2011.06.001
0891-8422/11/$ – see front matter © 2011 Elsevier Inc. All rights reserved.

podiatric.theclinics.com

the reader with a thorough and informative Arthroscopy of the Ankle and Foot edition of *Clinics in Podiatric Medicine and Surgery*.

Laurence G. Rubin, DPM
Private Practice, 3808 Hackamore Lane
Richmond, VA 23233, USA

E-mail address:
lgrubin@comcast.net

Practical Aspects of Foot and Ankle Arthroscopy

Meagan M. Jennings, DPM*, Samantha E. Bark, DPM

KEYWORDS

• Arthroscopy • Foot • Ankle

Arthroscopy of the foot and ankle, although sometimes technically challenging, is a useful tool for the foot and ankle surgeon. Burman[1] was the first to attempt arthroscopy of the ankle joint in 1931 and surmised that it was not a suitable joint for arthroscopy because of its narrow intra-articular space. With the development of smaller-diameter arthroscopes and improvements in joint distraction techniques, Watanabe[2] was the first to present a series of 28 ankle arthroscopes in 1972.

At present, arthroscopy is a valuable skill for the foot and ankle surgeon and is used not only to evaluate and treat intra-articular abnormalities but also for endoscopic and tendoscopic procedures.

INSTRUMENTATION

Requirements for arthroscopy are a light source, camera and monitor, arthroscope, and ingress of fluid. The arthroscope is essentially a telescope in a cannula that protects the scope and allows for controlled ingress and egress of fluid. The light source attaches to the scope and illuminates the joint using fiberoptic bundles. The bundles are coupled with a rod-lens system that carries reflected light images from the interior of the joint through the camera, and the image of the interior of the joint is projected on the monitor.

The arthroscope ranges in size from smaller than 1.5 mm in diameter to 7.3 mm; the larger the diameter of the scope, the larger the viewing surface, which increases exponentially (surface area $= \pi r^2$). A 4-mm-diameter scope is typically used for ankle arthroscopy (**Fig. 1**). The advent of wide-angled scopes has allowed the development of ankle and small joint arthroscopy. Traditional arthroscopes have the lens angled at 90° to the long axis of the scope. However, the smaller-diameter scopes are cut at 30° and 70° to the long axis of the scope, giving a larger viewing surface and improved

Disclosure: The authors have nothing to disclose.
Department of Podiatry, Palo Alto Medical Foundation, 701 East El Camino Real, Mountain View, CA 94040, USA
* Corresponding author.
E-mail address: Jenninm1@pamf.org

0891-8422/11/$ – see front matter © 2011 Elsevier Inc. All rights reserved.
podiatric.theclinics.com

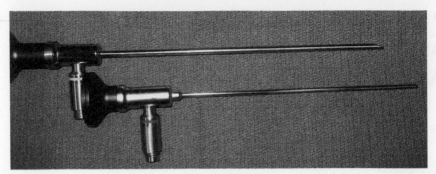

Fig. 1. The 4.0- and 2.7-mm arthroscopes are the most commonly used in foot and ankle arthroscopy.

visibility in these small spaces. The 30° and 70° scopes have different viewing fields. The 30° scope allows the arthroscopist a field of vision in line with the scope and 30° to the periphery, whereas the 70° scope allows a field of vision 70° to the periphery but not directly ahead (**Fig. 2**).

Hand Instruments

A variety of instruments have been made for arthroscopy. For ankle arthroscopy, instruments with a diameter less than 5 mm are ideal, and for smaller foot joints, a diameter less than 3 mm is ideal. The typical nonmotorized hand instruments available are probes, graspers, curettes, knives, osteotomes, gouges, punches, rongeurs, and magnetized rods (**Figs. 3–7**). Probes are often marked as a measuring device in 1- to 2-mm increments and also allow the size of lesions to be measured.

Power Instruments

Motorized instruments (cutters, shavers, and burrs/abraders) are often more efficient especially for debriding synovitis and fibrous bands as well as removing osteophytes. They include an aspiration component when attached to suction, which brings the tissue closer to the cutting edge of the instrument. There are various types of shavers including side cutting, open ended, and full radius. The side-cutting shaver has a small window that does not allow exposure to the blade's distal tip. These are the least aggressive of the power instruments. The open-ended shaver is the most aggressive and has the distal tip of the blade exposed. Probably the most commonly used is a combination of the 2 types, which is called a full-radius shaver. It has only partial exposure of the tip of the blade and the side-cutting window (**Figs. 8** and **9**). The full-radius shavers are either smooth (traditional type) or with incisors. The incisor types are either single or double incisor, meaning that both the barrel and the blade have teeth for a double incisor and only the blade has incisors on a single incisor. Typically, the power setting used is between 1500 and 3000 rpm. If the rotation of the blade is too fast, it will not allow the instrument to pull adequate tissue into the device.

Thermoablative Tools

Other tools available to the arthroscopic surgeon include arthroscopic radiofrequency wands and, to a lesser extent, holmium-YAG laser systems that can vaporize, shrink, coagulate, and even weld tissue. Although arthroscopic laser technology has been available for more than 15 years, it remains controversial because it is expensive, requires special training, and remains unproven regarding its benefits.[3] In recent

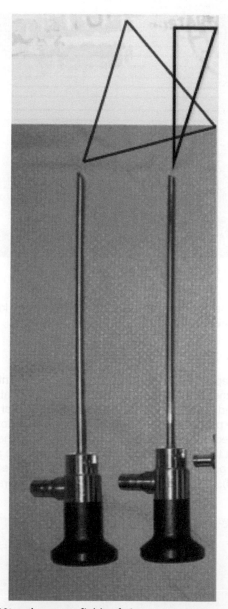

Fig. 2. The 70° versus 30° arthroscope fields of view.

years, radiofrequency wand technology has advanced significantly to effectively manage soft tissue abnormalities, especially in a cleanup role after the bulk of the soft tissue has been removed using a shaver or an ablator. The tips of the instruments vary in size to adapt to small-sized and medium-sized joints. Proper fluid management is important to regulate intra-articular temperature with these devices; this is combined with surgeon-controlled power adjustments to match tissue density and response to thermoablation. Some radiofrequency wands are aspirated to allow for suction application, which assists with fluid flow management, and to draw tissue

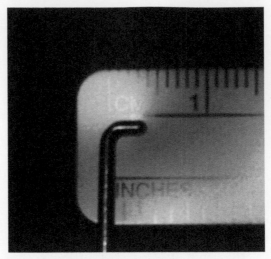

Fig. 3. Probes can often be used to judge lesion size.

into the wand tip. These suction types can also help to control intra-articular temperature because of the evacuation of heated fluid.

PATIENT POSITIONING

There are several acceptable positions for arthroscopy of the anterior ankle joint. The patient is placed supine, and the knee is either straight or bent over a knee stirrup, ramp, bump, or the end of the table (**Fig. 10**). Often, an ipsilateral hip bump is required to internally rotate the patient's leg. If an external ankle distractor is used, it is advantageous to use the knee stirrup for bending the hip and knee. The posterior ankle joint can be accessed with the patient placed supine if distraction is applied but also may be accessed through posterior portals when the patient is placed prone. For subtalar joint arthroscopy (STJ), the patient is typically placed in the lateral decubitus position.

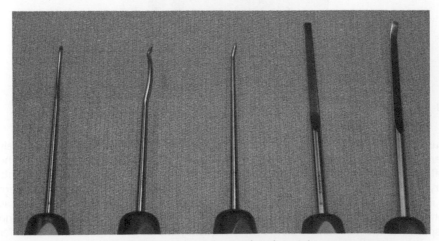

Fig. 4. Arthroscopy osteochondral picks and curved and straight osteotomes.

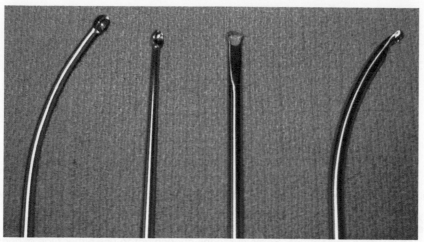

Fig. 5. Curettes can be cupped (left 2 images) and ring (right 2 images) as well as straight or curved to address lesions.

ANESTHESIA

The type of anesthesia is the surgeon's preference. Many arthroscopists elect for general anesthesia or spinal anesthesia for ease of joint manipulation and joint distraction.

Local anesthetic is also the surgeon's preference (see the "Joint Insufflation and Fluids" section).

HEMOSTASIS

Maintenance of a bloodless field during ankle arthroscopy is the surgeon's preference. The options are either tourniquet or pharmacologic hemostasis. The tourniquet may be placed at the thigh or calf. A sterile tourniquet could also be used at the proximal ankle. However, this can interfere with tissue mobilization when inflated. For pharmacologic hemostasis, epinephrine (1 mg/L) can be infused with the ingress fluid. If an

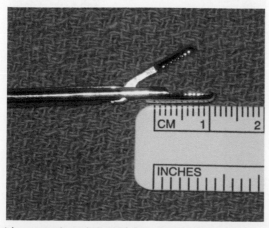

Fig. 6. A grasper with serrated teeth is useful to remove loose bodies and tissue.

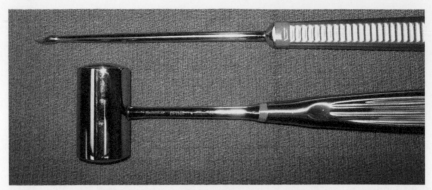

Fig. 7. A gouge has a scoop-like head and sharp leading edge to aid in osteophyte removal.

open procedure is anticipated after completion of arthroscopy, tourniquet time can be spared by using epinephrine. Some surgeons choose not to use either type of hemostasis and rely on joint distension. Intra-articular hemostasis can be performed with a thermoablative wand when necessary. If a tourniquet is used, it should be deflated before final closure of the portals and bandage placement for the assessment of hemostasis. If there is excessive intra-articular bleeding without major vessel injury, a closed suction drain may be placed through the portal into the joint.

JOINT DISTRACTION

Distraction of the joint is the surgeon's preference and may be necessary in cases with talar dome lesions located in the posterior half of the joint surface or other abnormality necessitating posterior ankle joint access through the anterior portals. Distraction

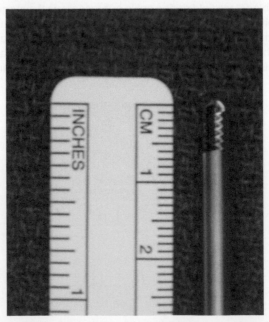

Fig. 8. Power shaver with double incisors of both the barrel and blade for grabbing tissue.

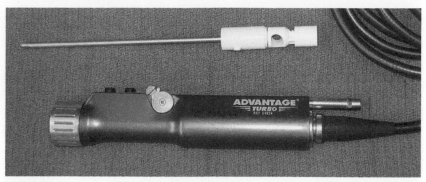

Fig. 9. Handpiece for power instrumentation. Shavers and burrs can be disposable or nondisposable.

allows the surgeon to pass the arthroscope and instruments between the articular surfaces without damaging the cartilage. There are invasive and noninvasive methods of physically pulling apart the joint surfaces. Invasive methods involve devices that directly engage bone, whereas noninvasive methods involve straps and bands. Simple noninvasive distraction can be achieved with gauze bandaging wrapped around the foot and ankle and applying distraction with weights or attaching to the surgeon's person who simply leans away from the patient (**Fig. 11**).[4,5] There are also commercially available noninvasive distraction straps that attach to the operating table. Countertraction with a knee stirrup is helpful in providing optimal traction with a noninvasive distraction device. Care must be taken to pad bony prominences and subcutaneous nerves when using the stirrup and the noninvasive joint distractor to help prevent neurapraxia as a result of compression forces.

Arthroscopy of the subtalar joint usually does not necessitate distraction. The capsular reflection typically provides enough room for instrumentation. Distraction of the first metatarsophalangeal joint can be helpful for joint visualization and can

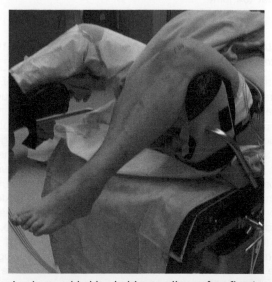

Fig. 10. Leg positioning in a padded leg holder to allow a free floating ankle.

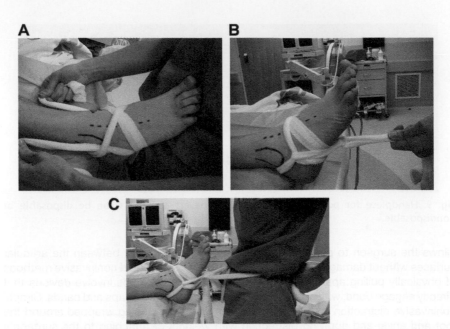

Fig. 11. (*A–C*) Demonstration of external ankle distraction using Kerlex gauze roll. Starting behind the heel with ends of the gauze in each hand, cross the 2 strands across the dorsum of the foot and then cross on the plantar surface of the foot (like a figure of 8). Place the 2 free ends back up through the most proximal straps (*A*) and then pull distally and tie under foot (*B*). A second roll can be placed through the bottom of the gauze foot strap and placed around the surgeon's waist. Then, the surgeon can distract by leaning backward as demonstrated in (*C*).

be achieved with a finger trap type noninvasive distractor attached to 2.3 to 6.8 kg (5–15 pounds) of distraction. Also, an invasive mini-rail external fixator can be used to distract the great toe joint.

TOPOGRAPHIC ANATOMY, PORTALS, AND ARTHROSCOPIC ANATOMY
Topographic Anatomy and Portals

The arthroscopic surgeon must have an excellent understanding of the topographic anatomy for accurate portal placement and avoidance of critical structures. Accurate portal placement aids in achieving the surgical goal and accessing most of the joint. For access of the posterior ankle from an anterior approach, if the portals are placed too high, it will be impossible to reach the posterior lesion. Some surgeons find it helpful to mark critical structures before portal development, including the tip of the lateral malleolus, medial malleolus, tibialis anterior tendon, and peroneus tertius tendon (which may be absent in some people). The intermediate dorsal cutaneous nerve is the most common structure injured during arthroscopy of the ankle because of its close proximity to the anterolateral portal. This structure can be mapped by plantar flexing the foot and the fourth toe, which places traction on the nerve, making it visible in many patients (**Fig. 12**). Because there are many variations of the vessels and nerves, it is imperative to use a proper technique of portal development (**Table 1**). Dorsiflexion of the ankle joint with one's thumb on the dome of the talus also helps to identify the anterior joint line and guide portal placement.

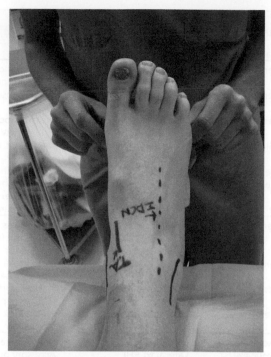

Fig. 12. Right ankle demonstrating intermediate dorsal cutaneous nerve and tibialis anterior.

In STJ, the most important topographic structure is the floor of the sinus tarsi. The entire surgery is keyed off this location and is critical for accurate portal placement. Palpatating the anterior beak of the calcaneus and sinus tarsi helps to identify portal placement. Another guide in STJ portal placement is to use 1 thumb breadth inferior and distal to the tip of the lateral malleolus (**Fig. 13**). The course of the sural nerve is important to understand in situations in which the middle portal or large-bore needles are placed to facilitate removal of air or outflow of fluid.

Arthroscopic Ankle Anatomy

The ankle joint is divided into 2 zones: the capsular reflection and the space between the articular surfaces of the talus, tibia, and fibula. The capsular reflection is the space between the capsule and the osteocartilaginous surfaces. Anteriorly, the capsular reflection contains a significant space, allowing for entry and manipulation of the arthroscope and instrumentation. The intra-articular space requires distraction or manipulation for passage of the arthroscope or other arthroscopic instruments.

The joint capsule and pericapsular ligaments define the capsular reflection of the ankle. The anterior capsular reflection is divided into anterior, lateral, and medial gutters. The anterior gutter is the space directly dorsal to the talar neck and anterior to the tibial surface. Recall that the anterior ankle joint capsule attaches to the anterior tibia 4 to 9 mm superior to the ankle joint line.[6] Several ankle ligaments can be visualized arthroscopically, including the deep deltoid, anterior talofibular, and anteroinferior tibiofibular ligaments. The posterior capsular reflection of the ankle has much less volume than the anterior aspect and is composed of the thick fibrous labrum of the posterior tibiofibular ligament, transverse ligament, and joint capsule. These thick

Table 1
Foot and ankle arthroscopic portals

Joint	Portal	Location	Comment
Ankle	Anteromedial	Between AT and medial malleolus	First portal developed, assess anterior pathology
	Anterolateral	Just lateral to peroneus tertius tendon	IDCN in close proximity
	Anterocentral	Between EHL and NV bundle	Accessory portal, high risk due to NV bundle
	Medial midline[16]	Between EHL and TA	Average of 11 mm from NV bundle[16]
	Posteromedial	Medial to TA	Close proximity to NV bundle
	Posterolateral	Lateral to TA	Accessible by switch stick maneuver
	Split TA	Through middle of TA	Causes trauma to TA
Subtalar	Anterolateral	Floor of sinus tarsi	Main access portal for anterior, lateral gutter and posterior access
	Lateral central	Lateral to anterolateral portal	Close proximity to sural nerve, used for fluid egress
	Accessory anterior	Just above anterolateral portal	Stacked portal technique for anterior pathology
	Posterolateral	Lateral to TA	Switch stick accessibility, posterior pathology
First MTPJ	Dorsomedial	Medial to EHL	Utility portal
	Dorsolateral	Lateral to EHL	Accessory portal

Abbreviations: AT, anterior tibial tendon; EHL, extensor hallucis longus; IDCN, intermediate dorsal cutaneous nerve; MTPJ, metatarsophalangeal joint; NV, neurovascular; TA, Achilles tendon.

tissues prevent distension of the capsule and limit the space available for manipulation of the arthroscope and instrumentation. Just inferior to the posterior ankle, the capsular recess is the posterior facet of the subtalar joint.

The posterior capsular reflection of the posterior facet of the subtalar joint is large and can be accessed from a posterolateral approach located lateral to the Achilles tendon. The anterior portion of the posterior facet is less amply endowed with space, yet it is easily navigated by the floor of the sinus tarsi and the firm nature of the interosseous talocalcaneal ligament, which marks the deep anterior frontier of the joint. The lateral gutter of the subtalar joint is accessible and deep to the tip of the fibula, calcaneofibular ligament, and peroneal tendons. The instrumentation can run along the calcaneal side of the posterior facet of the subtalar joint. When traversing the lateral gutter, it is possible to observe the posterior facet and the saddle centrally. The posterior talofibular ligament can be visualized parallel to the posterior half of the posterior facet and terminating at the posterior process.

The capsular reflection of the great toe joint is present in significant variance of volume on the dorsal aspect of the joint. Degenerative changes associated with hallux limitus and hallux valgus frequently obscure the capsular reflection.

JOINT INSUFFLATION AND FLUIDS

Once appropriate anesthesia is achieved and a sterile field created, the joint capsule is distended with the insufflation of fluid. Distension of the joint before portal development has several benefits. It allows the surgeon to accurately place the portals based on the path of the needle into the joint and allows for easier placement of the blunt

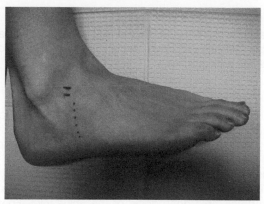

Fig. 13. Demonstration of the placement of standard anterior lateral STJ portal placement on the floor of the sinus tarsi. Dotted line represents the calcaneocuboid joint.

trocar through a taught joint capsule as opposed to through a flimsy loose layer of soft tissue. Joint distension is necessary for visualization, which is imperative for arthroscopy, and may be easier to maintain if achieved before portal development. When the joint is sufficiently distended (a typical volume of 15–40 mL), the surgeon may notice a palpable bubble of distended capsule and slight dorsiflexion of the ankle as the end of distention of the capsule is achieved.

There are many options of fluids for joint insufflation. Many surgeons insufflate with a local anesthetic with or without epinephrine before beginning the procedure but only after all anatomic landmarks have been assessed to avoid movement of these marks with joint distention. Some surgeons use normal saline (NS) or lactated Ringer (LR) solution and inject local anesthetic only at the end of the procedure. NS and LR are the most commonly used for maintenance of distention. LR solution is more closely related to a physiologic milieu than NS and commonly readily available at a cost comparable with that of NS.[7–9]

Maintenance of distension is a careful balancing act between ingress and egress of fluid into the joint delivered by either gravity flow or active pump. Ingress occurs through the cannula of the arthroscope and egress along the surface of the instruments inserted in the portals. If there is not enough ingress, which can occur with arthroscopes of diameter less than 4 mm, extra cannulas may be placed. Likewise, if sufficient egress is not achieved, placing an 18-gauge needle into the joint will suffice for egress of fluid from the joint. This balancing act requires careful attention from the surgeon throughout the procedure. There is the potential for fluid to accumulate in the periarticular soft tissues, which should be monitored by the surgeons and assistants. The use of a fluid ingress pump may increase the potential for extravasation if the pressure is too high. Although there are at present no reports of morbidity associated with fluid extravasation during ankle arthroscopy, compartment syndrome has been reported after knee arthroscopy.[10]

Intra-articular injection of local anesthetics after completion of the arthroscopic procedure is common practice. Recent publications demonstrate cartilage toxicity (chondrocyte death) with prolonged exposure to lidocaine and bupivacaine.[11–15] Even adjusting the pH of the local anesthetic has no effect on the toxic effects on cartilage.[13] Ropivacaine has been reported to have less toxicity than bupivacaine in human chondrocytes and has become the drug of choice for intra-articular injections for many surgeons.[15]

SUMMARY

Arthroscopy is a valuable skill for the foot and ankle surgeon's armamentarium. With practice, various abnormalities may be treated arthroscopically, avoiding the morbidity from large incisions and arthrotomies.

REFERENCES

1. Burman MS. Arthroscopy of direct visualization of joints. An experimental cadaver study. J Bone Joint Surg 1931;13:669–95.
2. Watanabe M. Selfoc arthroscope (Watanabe no 24 arthroscopes) monograph. Tokyo: Teishin Hospital; 1972.
3. Brillhart AT. Lasers in arthroscopic surgery [letter]. Arthroscopy 1991;7:411–2.
4. Miyamoto W, Takao M, Komatu F, et al. Technique tip: the bandage distraction technique for arthroscopic arthrodesis of the ankle joint. Foot Ankle Int 2008; 29:251–3.
5. Yates CK, Grana WA. A simple distraction technique for ankle arthroscopy. Arthroscopy 1988;4:103–5.
6. Tol JL, van Dijk CN. Etiology of the anterior ankle impingement syndrome: a descriptive anatomical study. Foot Ankle Int 2004;25(6):382–6.
7. Reagan BF, McInerny VK, Treadwell BV, et al. Irrigating solutions for arthroscopy. A metabolic study. J Bone Joint Surg Am 1983;65:629–31.
8. Shinjo H, Nakata K, Shino K, et al. Effect of irrigation solutions for arthroscopic surgery on intraarticular tissue: comparison in human meniscus-derived primary cell culture between lactate Ringer's solution and saline solution. J Orthop Res 2002;20:1305–10.
9. Yang CY, Cheng SC, Shen CL. Effect of irrigation fluid on the articular cartilage: a scanning electron microscope study. Arthroscopy 1993;9:425–30.
10. Kaper BP, Carr CF, Shirreffs TG. Compartments syndrome after arthroscopic surgery of the knee. A report of two cases managed non-operatively. Am J Sports Med 1997;25(1):123–5.
11. Chu CR, Izzo NJ, Coyle CH, et al. The in vitro effects of bupivacaine on articular chondrocytes. J Bone Joint Surg Br 2008;90:814–20.
12. Chu CR, Izzo NJ, Papas NE, et al. In vitro exposure to 0.5% bupivacaine is cyto-toxic to bovine articular chondrocytes. Arthroscopy 2006;22:693–9.
13. Karpie JC, Chu CR. Lidocaine exhibits dose- and time-dependent cytotoxic effects on bovine articular chondrocytes in vitro. Am J Sports Med 2007;35: 1621–7.
14. Nole R, Munson NM, Fulkerson JP. Bupivacaine and saline effects on articular cartilage. Arthroscopy 1985;1:123–7.
15. Piper SL, Kim HT. Comparison of ropivacaine and bupivacaine toxicity in human articular chondrocytes. J Bone Joint Surg Am 2008;90:986–91.
16. Buckingham RA, Winson IG, Kelly AJ. An anatomical study of a new portal for ankle arthroscopy. J Bone Joint Surg Br 1997;79(4):650–2.

Preoperative Evaluation and Testing for Arthroscopy

Sean T. Grambart, DPM[a], Benjamin D. Overley Jr, DPM[b]

KEYWORDS

- Arthroscopy • Ankle surgery • Preoperative planning
- Ankle imaging

Although reports of arthroscopic procedures have dated back to the 19th century, in 1918, Kenji Takagi designed the first arthroscope and is regarded as the father of modern arthroscopy. The initial foundation of arthroscopy is based on arthroscopic procedures on the knee. In the 1970s, Watanabe reported on the first attempts at ankle arthroscopy. Technological advancement with modern arthroscopes and instrumentation, as well as well-designed, hands-on instructional courses, has not only made ankle arthroscopy a popular and highly successful procedure, but has expanded the surgical procedures to other joints and tendons of the foot and ankle.

INDICATIONS

Understanding when to proceed with an arthroscopy of the ankle and foot can at times be difficult. Before proceeding with any arthroscopy, a complete understanding of the intra-articular and extra-articular structures is essential to a positive surgical outcome. The knowledge of these structures and their topographic anatomy in and about the ankle and foot will assist the surgeon in appropriately advised surgical intervention, as well as in avoiding iatrogenic pitfalls.

Currently, there are no *absolute* contraindications for arthroscopy of the ankle.[1] However, there are some relative contraindications, such as patients with compromised circulation or patients with comorbid medical issues.

Glazebrook and colleagues[1] reported "that the basis for arthroscopy for indications such as ankle instability, septic arthritis, arthrofibrosis, removal of loose bodies or ankle arthritis in the absence of bony impingement lacked sufficient evidence based

[a] Department of Surgery, Carle Physician Group, 1802 South Mattis Avenue, Champaign, IL 61821, USA
[b] The Sports Medicine Institute, 1601 Medical Drive, Pottstown, PA 19464
E-mail address: Sean.Grambart@carle.com

Clin Podiatr Med Surg 28 (2011) 453–467
doi:10.1016/j.cpm.2011.04.007
0891-8422/11/$ – see front matter © 2011 Elsevier Inc. All rights reserved.

support." Conversely, they reported that, "preparative ankle arthrodesis approaches, osteochondral lesion repairs and treatment of ankle impingement syndromes were fairly supported as indications." For the purpose of simplification, relative indications for ankle arthroscopy can be divided into 3 distinct surgical categories based on the desired final outcome for the procedure:

1. Arthroscopic ankle survey
2. Arthroscopic reparative ankle surgery
3. Arthroscopic ablative ankle surgery.

Arthroscopic survey should be considered when preoperative assessment of the ankle joint does not yield a confirmative diagnosis via clinical, physical, or diagnostic testing. Arthroscopic survey in the ankle joint may also be desired as a precursor to anticipated reparative arthroscopic procedures as well.

Indications for an ankle arthroscopic survey include lavage for septic joint with survey, syndesmotic analysis, preemptive assessment of joint before an intended open repair, assessment of poorly placed internal or external fixation hardware, and arthroscopic biopsy. With respect to arthroscopic survey, the scope of the procedure is relatively narrow, as one would expect with any operative survey. Surveys may be performed after an examination under anesthesia with mortise and Broden's views of the ankle under image intensification before a formal repair of the lateral ligament and retinacular structures or "Brostrom" (modified or true) repair for ankle joint instability. An arthroscopic survey may also be beneficial as a diagnostic tool when infection is suspected. "Ankle joint surveys performed to inspect and treat septic ankle joints have also been successful as a treatment modality though there is a paucity of literature to support this technique."[1,2] The success of this approach may be directly related to the physiologic lavage and reduction of a pathologic microorganism count more so than the topical introduction of antibiotic-rich saline.

Reparative arthroscopy may be indicated when preoperative assessment examinations are relatively conclusive for an underlying pathology via clinical, physical, or diagnostic findings. Simply put, this is a surgical "search and remove/repair" approach to ankle arthroscopy. Reparative indications include synovectomy, ligament repair, osteochondral defect repair, capsular thermocautery, intra-articular fracture reduction, arthrofibrosis, impingement syndromes (either soft tissue or osseous), and os trigonum resection.

Another parameter in the surgical decision-making process as to whether an open repair versus an arthroscopic procedure is better indicated can be made on realization of the constraints of an arthroscopic approach to the ankle joint. Studies have shown that patients with bony or soft tissue impingements tend to do better with smaller focal impingements and a lack of significant osteoarthritis.[1,3,4] This consideration is an important one if solely for the purpose of open treatment consent and appropriate instrumentation being available at time of surgery.

If there is definitive presence of an osteochondral defect (OCD),[1,5] a reparative arthroscopic approach may be attempted to reduce the defect and relieve pain.[1,4,6] However, careful consideration should be given to the location of the defect. The location of the lesion may play a significant role in the postoperative outcome of the repair. A talar dome defect or tibial plafond defect may respond better to arthroscopic repair versus a shoulder defect of the talus or a medial/lateral gutter defect. Kelberine and Frank compared anterolateral OCD repair versus posteromedial repair and reported that the anterolateral group had significantly better results (89%) versus the posteromedial study group (63%) with regard to patient improvement and overall satisfaction.[5] This is a statistically significant finding when transposed against the long-accepted notion that anterolateral OCD repair should not be attempted owing to the lack of improvement and the location of the lesion. It should also be noted that posteromedial defects are commonly associated with plantarflexion/inversion sprains, whereas anterolateral lesions are more commonly a result of a dorsiflexion/inversion injury. These 2 common defects also differ in their presentations from an arthroscopic appearance. Anterolateral lesions are typically "wafer" shaped and relatively superficial, whereas posteromedial lesions are typically more "cup" shaped, indicating a deeper injury. In addition, the proximity of anterolateral OCDs to structures that may be contributing pain sources may also add to the higher postoperative scores by easier access to these structures during the defect repair.[5,6] Conversely, posteromedial lesions may be difficult to access at the time of surgery and may require malleolar osteotomy or a posteromedial approach depending on the size of the lesion and its location. For example, an anterolateral soft tissue impingement by traumatic thickening of Bassett's ligament can be repaired concomitantly during the repair of an anterolateral OCD.

Relatively new indications for ankle arthroscopy are always emerging that include joint debridement for arthrodesis, management of septic joints, and aid in fracture reduction. Thermocautery or "capsular shrinkage procedures," intra-articular fracture reduction, and ankle arthrodesis procedures are relatively new and are gaining support as indications for ankle arthroscopy. In cases of arthroscopic thermocautery for ankle joint instability, Berlet and colleagues[7] and Hyer and Vancourt[8] reported good results with lateral ankle stability using thermocautery with lateral ankle gutter debridement.

Intra-articular open reduction of fractures via ankle arthroscopy has also become more popular in recent years both intraoperatively and postoperatively.[1,3,9] During an open reduction of an intra-articular fracture of the ankle joint complex (tibia, talus, and fibula), arthroscopy can be used to verify anatomic reduction of the joint surfaces with debridement of any cartilage defects that may be present. Postoperatively, if painful hardware becomes an issue, arthroscopy also can be performed with hardware removal as an adjunctive procedure to enhance postoperative results in the presence of minimal posttraumatic arthritis.[3]

Surgical ablative arthroscopy is indicated when the procedure is used as a surgical "means to an end" to a more comprehensive procedure, such as joint preparation for ankle joint arthrodesis. The increased usage of this technique to perform a "minimally invasive" arthrodesis procedure versus a traditional open ankle arthrodesis has been fairly well supported by current literature.[1,10–12] Good results have been demonstrated with use of this technique.[1,10,11] This minimal approach may be gaining acceptance because of the reduction in tourniquet time and wound morbidity associated with traditional open procedures.[1]

In summary, there are no accepted, absolute indications for ankle and foot arthroscopy. However, besides the aforementioned common indications for arthroscopy, adapted indications have expanded its usefulness as an adjunct procedure to treat infection, fracture, or arthrodesis and is a vital surgical procedure to treat ankle joint disorders.

PATIENT HISTORY AND THE PHYSICAL EXAMINATION

When evaluating a patient for arthroscopic surgery, a thorough and complete history of the patient's complaints must be obtained. The patient's histories of present illness, and past medical and surgical histories are essential to establishing a conclusive diagnosis. For example, a patient with a history of multiple ankle sprains may present with pain owing to instability.

The physical examination, however, will most undoubtedly yield the greatest diagnostic benefit of any test. Careful, sequential examination of the ankle joint and its bony and soft tissue structures along with diagnostic testing and a thorough history will provide the examiner with the necessary information to make an informative diagnosis.

Examiners should take a systematic, "around-the-world" approach to examining the ankle joint. This approach is performed at the farthest point from the suspected pain foci and progresses to the foci in both directions in a circumferential matter. When performed repeatedly, the examiner will develop a unique proficiency for recognizing certain ankle pathologies. All of the bony and soft tissue structures that pass the ankle joint should be palpated as well as palpation of the joint line and its corresponding landmarks. By working in a continuous manner about the ankle joint, the examiner will be able to eliminate redundancies (referred pain) in presentation as well as adding to the efficiency of the examination. Patients should be sitting up on an examination chair or table with the lower extremities in open chain attitude (heels free) for an accurate physical examination. Some examples of palpation tests are shown in **Figs. 1 to 6**.

While performing palpation of any structure of or surrounding the ankle joint, it is imperative to simultaneously flex, rotate, and circumduct the ankle joint. For instance, pain from anterolateral impingement may be vague if the anterolateral joint line is palpated solely. However, with maximum ankle joint dorsiflexion, a more profound pain response may be elicited, providing the examiner with a better-defined diagnosis.

For a test of the sinus tarsi and subtalar joint (see **Fig. 6**), the foot should be plantarflexed and inverted slightly to allow for better feel on the examiner's part.

The "crossover exam" (see **Fig. 3**) is an essential examination for diagnosing an injury to the ATFL (anterior talofibular ligament). In this author's opinion, it is more reliable then the more widely used "squeeze test." The squeeze test may elicit pain but this may be a result of several factors, such as hemarthrosis redirection or loading of an insufficiency fracture of the malleoli, whereas the crossover examination places the patient's symptomatic ankle above the asymptomatic one and allows the examiner to gently palpate the distal tibiofibular complex. The examiner should attempt to spread the tibia and fibula apart at their most distal attachments. A positive response from this is usually indicative of syndesmotic injury (sprain or tear).

In conclusion, the history and physical examination components of the patient encounter will provide the most vital information for the examiner as to the severity and location of the patient's pain. The careful examiner will clinically correlate any test results with the history and physical findings to arrive at an informed differential diagnosis.

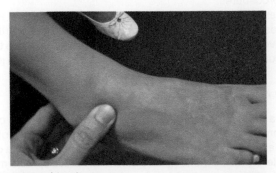

Fig. 1. Test for anterolateral impingement.

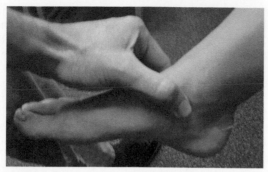

Fig. 2. Test for medial lateral ankle gutter impingement.

IMAGING FOR ARTHROSCOPY
Soft Tissue Pathology

Soft tissue pathology that is commonly treated with arthroscopy includes synovitis, impingement syndromes, and a multitude of soft tissue pathology. Although radiographs are typically negative for soft tissue pathology, they are important in the initial evaluation to rule out osseous pathology, such as fractures and joint space degeneration. Computed tomography (CT) scans are not recommended if the initial radiographs are negative for osseous pathology; however, CT scans can be used if initial radiographs show irregularity along the medial and lateral radiographs. Increased irregularity along the lateral gutter has been shown to correspond to a meniscoid lesion and an extensive fibrotic reactive tissue.[13]

Although Ferkel and colleagues[14,15] have concluded that magnetic resonance imaging (MRI) was the most effective diagnostic screening test, other studies have questioned the reliability of MRI in diagnosing ankle impingement. In a study of 22 athletes with suspected anterolateral impingement, Liu and colleagues[16] showed that MRI had a sensitivity and specificity of 39% and 50% respectively, whereas clinical examination had a sensitivity of 94% and specificity of 75%, using arthroscopy as the gold standard. With suspected ankle impingement pathology, MRI can be effective by identifying other pathology that can also be present.[17]

The use of intravenous contrast in enhancing vascularized soft tissue pathology is often used for indirect MRI arthrography. Vascularized scar tissue and synovium will

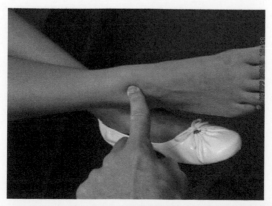

Fig. 3. "Crossover" examination for syndesmotic/"high ankle sprain."

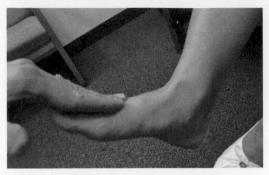

Fig. 4. Dorsiflexion test for retinacular/anterior tibial tendon pain.

undergo contrast enhancement, whereas avascular soft tissue pathology such as meniscoid bodies may not enhance. Given that many causes of impingement may be avascular lesions, Haller and associates[18] showed that indirect MRI arthrography may be less accurate than conventional MR imaging. Direct MR arthrography is another modality for attempting to enhance soft tissue pathology.[19] Robinson and colleagues[19] prospectively performed MR arthrography to assess the anterolateral gutter/recess in 32 patients. All 12 patients with clinical evidence of anterolateral impingement and an abnormal anterolateral gutter recess at arthroscopy demonstrated either focal or irregular nodular soft tissue thickening in the anterolateral gutter at MR arthrography.

The authors used conventional MRI for evaluating structures surrounding the ankle joint rather than intra-articular soft tissue pathology. Diagnostic injections, which will be discussed later, are the author's preferred method for determining the amount of pain from intra-articular pathology. Arthroscopy is then used for both diagnostic and therapeutic purposes.

Bony Impingement and Loose Bodies

Bony impingement can typically be observed with standard radiographs. Lateral ankle views are the most helpful (**Fig. 7**). Stress views can be used as well. CT scans can aid with identifying the exact location, size, and condition of the articular surface surrounding the osseous impingement (**Fig. 8**). Conventional MRI is a useful tool when evaluating the location and size of the bony impingement or loose bodies

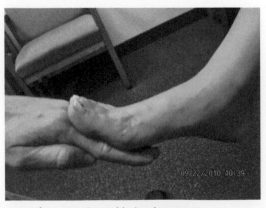

Fig. 5. Plantarflexion test for posterior ankle impingement.

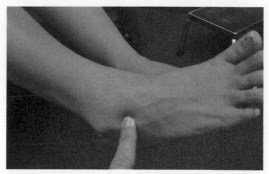

Fig. 6. Test for sinus tarsi/subtalar joint pathology.

(**Fig. 9**). With long-standing symptoms, an MRI can be useful in determining osteo-chondral pathology as well.

Osteochondral Lesions

Standard weight-bearing radiographs are indicated as the initial radiographic study for suspected osteochondral lesions. These typically present as a radiopaque lesion most commonly on the medial and lateral shoulders of the talus (**Fig. 10**). Unfortunately,

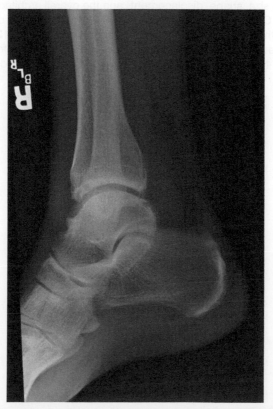

Fig. 7. Lateral radiograph of anterior ankle impingement.

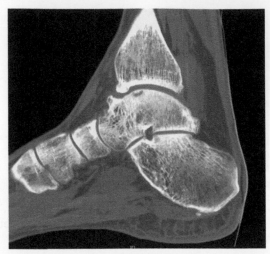

Fig. 8. Sagittal CT scan of tibiotalar osseous impingement.

a large percentage of osteochondral lesions, up to 50%, may not be visible on standard radiographs and radiographs do not assess the condition of the cartilage.[20–23]

CT scans also lack the ability to assess the articular cartilage, but have the advantage in evaluating size, shape, displacement, and the overall architecture of the bone injury (**Fig. 11**).[14] CT scans seem to be useful in evaluating acute, displaced osteochondral injuries that are initially diagnosed with radiographs (**Fig. 12**).

MRI currently seems to be the advanced imaging option of choice for osteochondral lesions (**Fig. 13**). Numerous classification systems for osteochondral lesions have

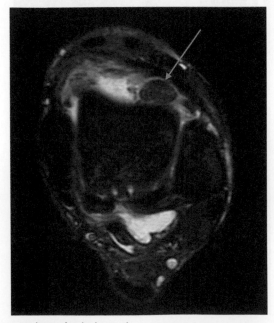

Fig. 9. Anterior osseous loose body (*arrow*).

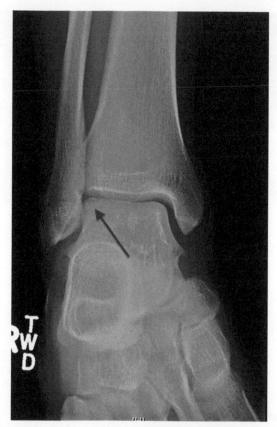

Fig. 10. Ankle radiograph of talar osteochondral lesion (*arrow*).

been developed using MRI.[21,24–27] Conventional MRIs evaluate the cartilage, sub-chondral bone, cancellous bone, and adjacent soft tissue structures while not exposing the patient to radiation.[28,29] MRI seems to correlate closely with arthro-scopic findings, but can overestimate the severity of the bone injury.[15,26]

Diagnostic Injections

Diagnostic injections are extremely useful for both the patient and the surgeon. Most patients will present with generalized "pain" when they present to the office. Injury to the osseous and soft tissue structures around joints will often be a vague pain and the patient may have difficulties pinpointing the exact location of the pain. Diagnostic intra-articular injections help the surgeon rule in or out joint pathology. Obviously this is helpful in determining if arthroscopy will be helpful or not. The other advantage is the patient can potentially see the amount of pain relief the arthroscopic procedure will give. Indications for diagnostic injections include chronic pain in the joint with advanced imaging studies showing no defined pathology and advanced imaging showing multiple areas of pathology, and also for patients who would like to see how much pain is coming from the joint.

Ankle Injection Technique

The theory behind the ankle injection technique is explained to the patient so the patient understands that this is a diagnostic injection and that once the local

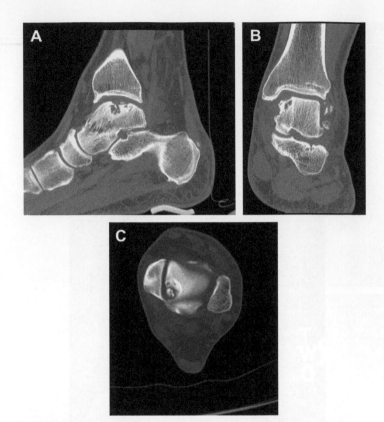

Fig. 11. (*A*) Sagittal CT OCD. (*B*) Coronal CT OCD. (*C*) Axial CT OCD.

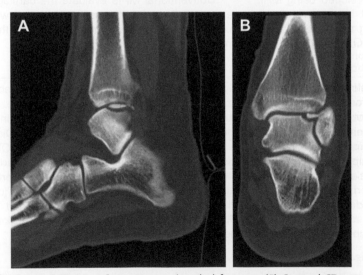

Fig. 12. (*A*) Sagittal CT scan of acute osteochondral fracture. (*B*) Coronal CT scan of acute osteochondral fracture.

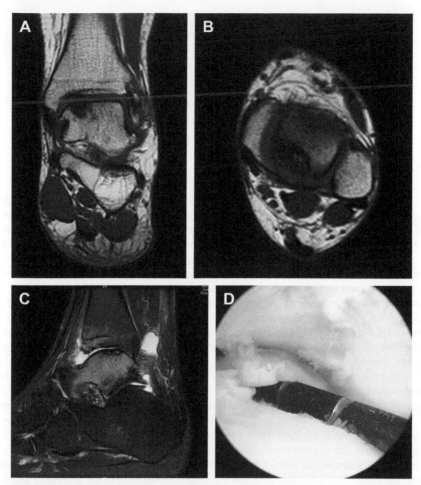

Fig. 13. (*A*) Coronal MRI of an osteochondral lesion. (*B*) Transverse MRI of an osteochondral lesion. (*C*) Sagittal MRI of an osteochondral lesion. (*D*) Corresponding arthroscopy of an osteochondral lesion.

anesthetic wears off, in a couple of hours, the pain will likely recur or may be slightly worse for a period of time. Risks are discussed such as the low risk of infection, hemarthrosis, and soft tissue and cartilage damage.

It is helpful to mark out the anatomic landmarks similar to starting an ankle arthroscopy (**Fig. 14**). The injection is approached from the anteromedial aspect. The tip of the medial malleolus and the medial aspect of the tibialis anterior tendon is marked. With the thumb held on the anterior ankle, the patient moves the ankle joint into plantarflexion and dorsiflexion. A mark is made slightly superior to where the surgeon's thumb feels the dorsal aspect of the neck of the talus on dorsiflexion. A line is drawn to connect the tip of the medial malleolus with the anterior ankle joint line mark. This is the approximate level of the ankle joint. The site for the injection is along the line medial to the tibialis anterior tendon.

The planned injection site is prepped with betadine (**Fig. 15**). Typically a 3-mL mixture of 1% lidocaine and 0.25% marcaine in a 50:50 ratio is used. The needle should be inserted in a posterior-lateral direction (**Fig. 16**). Ideally, the needle should

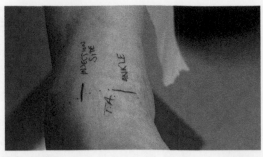

Fig. 14. Anteromedial injection site.

"fall" into the ankle joint. Once the needle is into the ankle, the local anesthetic is infiltrated in a slow, constant manner. Patients should feel pressure and have minimal pain. Once the injection is complete, the patient is encouraged to perform activities that typically cause discomfort in the ankle. Be sure to tell the patient that when the local anesthetic wears off, there will be increased discomfort in the ankle as a result of the activity. While the local anesthetic is in place, the patient needs to quantify the amount of pain relief in the ankle joint and contact the surgeon's office.

There is some controversy regarding the interaction of local anesthetic and its affects on chondrocytes. Bupivacaine has been found to be potentially harmful to chondrocytes in vitro.[30–32] Intra-articular injection of bupivacaine is the primary means of chondrocyte damage. The loss of articular cartilage as a result of lysis of the matrix and cells, known as chondrolysis, has been reported in the shoulder.[33] In vitro studies support the theory that chondrocyte necrosis may contribute to the rapid occurrence of chondrolysis with the use of bupivacaine.[34,35] Many of the theories suggest that the chondrolysis is dependent upon the time and dose of exposure to the local anesthetic. Chu and colleagues[30] reported on the in vitro effects of a single injection of saline or bupivacaine into a stifle joint in a rat model using a single injection of mono-iodoacetate into the contralateral stifle joint as the control. The results showed that the group with a single injection of bupivacaine showed reduced chondrocyte density without cartilage loss 6 months after the injection. As expected, the effects of bupivacaine were much milder than the injection of mono-iodoacetate in the control group, which caused chondrolysis at 6 months. The investigators concluded that a single intra-articular injection of bupivacaine has subtle effects on the articular cartilage and that the clinical effects would likely be difficult to detect. At this point, there is inconclusive evidence to make any definitive conclusion as to whether or not to use bupivacaine for intra-articular injections.

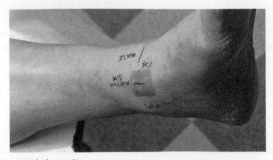

Fig. 15. Injection site with betadine.

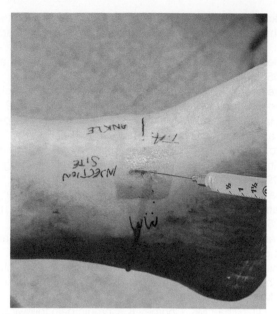

Fig. 16. Injection aiming toward the lateral malleolus.

SUMMARY

Proper preoperative planning will ensure that the correct surgical procedure is selected. Although most surgeons can determine the correct diagnosis and treatment options for the patient based on the subjective and objective examinations, advanced imaging and diagnostic injections are useful tools in difficult cases.

REFERENCES

1. Glazebrook MA, Ganapathy V, Bridge MA, et al. Evidence-based indications for ankle arthroscopy. Arthroscopy 2009;25(12):1478–90.
2. Vispo Seara JL, Barthel T, Schmitz H, et al. Arthroscopic treatment of septic joints: prognostic factors. Arch Orthop Trauma Surg 2002;122(4):204–11.
3. van Dijk CN, Verhagen RA, Tol JL. Arthroscopy for problems after ankle fracture. J Bone Joint Surg Br 1997;79(2):280–4.
4. Kim SH, Ha KI. Arthroscopic treatment for impingement of the anterolateral soft tissues of the ankle. J Bone Joint Surg Br 2000;82(7):1019–21.
5. Kelberine F, Frank A. Arthroscopic treatment of osteochondral lesions of the talar dome: a retrospective study of 48 cases. Arthroscopy 1999;15(1):77–84.
6. Schimmer RC, Dick W, Hintermann B. The role of ankle arthroscopy in the treatment strategies of osteochondritis dissecans lesions of the talus. Foot Ankle Int 2001;22(11):895–900.
7. Berlet GC, Saar WE, Ryan A, et al. Thermal-assisted capsular modification for functional ankle instability. Foot Ankle Clin 2002;7(3):567–76, ix.
8. Hyer CF, Vancourt R. Arthroscopic repair of lateral ankle instability by using the thermal-assisted capsular shift procedure: a review of 4 cases. J Foot Ankle Surg 2004;43(2):104–9.

9. Ono A, Nishikawa S, Nagao A, et al. Arthroscopically assisted treatment of ankle fractures: arthroscopic findings and surgical outcomes. Arthroscopy 2004;20(6): 627–31.

10. Ferkel RD, Hewitt M. Long-term results of arthroscopic ankle arthrodesis. Foot Ankle Int 2005;26(4):275–80.

11. Jerosch J, Steinbeck J, Schroder M, et al. Arthroscopically assisted arthrodesis of the ankle joint. Arch Orthop Trauma Surg 1996;115(3–4):182–9.

12. O'Brien TS, Hart TS, Shereff MJ, et al. Open versus arthroscopic ankle arthrodesis: a comparative study. Foot Ankle Int 1999;20(6):368–74.

13. Hauger O, Moinard M, Lasalarie JC, et al. Anterolateral compartment of the ankle in the lateral impingement syndrome: appearance on CT arthrography. AJR Am J Roentgenol 1999;173(3):685–90.

14. Ferkel RD, Flannigan BD, Elkins BS. Magnetic resonance imaging of the foot and ankle: correlation of normal anatomy with pathologic conditions. Foot Ankle 1991; 11(5):289–305.

15. Ferkel RD, Karzel RP, Del Pizzo W, et al. Arthroscopic treatment of anterolateral impingement of the ankle. Am J Sports Med 1991;19(5):440–6.

16. Liu SH, Nuccion SL, Finerman G. Diagnosis of anterolateral ankle impingement. Comparison between magnetic resonance imaging and clinical examination. Am J Sports Med 1997;25(3):389–93.

17. Ogilvie-Harris DJ, Gilbart MK, Chorney K. Chronic pain following ankle sprains in athletes: the role of arthroscopic surgery. Arthroscopy 1997;13(5):564–74.

18. Haller J, Bernt R, Seeger T, et al. MR-imaging of anterior tibiotalar impingement syndrome: agreement, sensitivity and specificity of MR-imaging and indirect MR-arthrography. Eur J Radiol 2006;58(3):450–60.

19. Robinson P, White LM, Salonen DC, et al. Anterolateral ankle impingement: MR arthrographic assessment of the anterolateral recess. Radiology 2001;221(1): 186–90.

20. Flick AB, Gould N. Osteochondritis dissecans of the talus (transchondral fractures of the talus): review of the literature and new surgical approach for medial dome lesions. Foot Ankle 1985;5(4):165–85.

21. Hepple S, Winson IG, Glew D. Osteochondral lesions of the talus: a revised classification. Foot Ankle Int 1999;20(12):789–93.

22. Loomer R, Fisher C, Lloyd-Smith R, et al. Osteochondral lesions of the talus. Am J Sports Med 1993;21(1):13–9.

23. Verhagen RA, Maas M, Dijkgraaf MG, et al. Prospective study on diagnostic strategies in osteochondral lesions of the talus. Is MRI superior to helical CT? J Bone Joint Surg Br 2005;87(1):41–6.

24. Anderson IF, Crichton KJ, Grattan-Smith T, et al. Osteochondral fractures of the dome of the talus. J Bone Joint Surg Am 1989;71(8):1143–52.

25. Dipaola JD, Nelson DW, Colville MR. Characterizing osteochondral lesions by magnetic resonance imaging. Arthroscopy 1991;7(1):101–4.

26. Mintz DN, Tashjian GS, Connell DA, et al. Osteochondral lesions of the talus: a new magnetic resonance grading system with arthroscopic correlation. Arthroscopy 2003;19(4):353–9.

27. Taranow WS, Bisignani GA, Towers JD, et al. Retrograde drilling of osteochondral lesions of the medial talar dome. Foot Ankle Int 1999;20(8):474–80.

28. Wells D, Oloff-Solomon J. Radiographic evaluation of transchondral dome fractures of the talus. J Foot Surg 1987;26(3):186–93.

29. Yulish BS, Mulopulos GP, Goodfellow DB, et al. MR imaging of osteochondral lesions of talus. J Comput Assist Tomogr 1987;11(2):296–301.

30. Chu CR, Coyle CH, Chu CT, et al. In vivo effects of single intra-articular injection of 0.5% bupivacaine on articular cartilage. J Bone Joint Surg Am 2010;92(3): 599–608.
31. Chu CR, Izzo NJ, Papas NE, et al. In vitro exposure to 0.5% bupivacaine is cytotoxic to bovine articular chondrocytes. Arthroscopy 2006;22(7):693–9.
32. Piper SL, Kim HT. Comparison of ropivacaine and bupivacaine toxicity in human articular chondrocytes. J Bone Joint Surg Am 2008;90(5):986–91.
33. Hansen BP, Beck CL, Beck EP, et al. Postarthroscopic glenohumeral chondrolysis. Am J Sports Med 2007;35(10):1628–34.
34. Chu CR, Izzo NJ, Coyle CH, et al. The in vitro effects of bupivacaine on articular chondrocytes. J Bone Joint Surg Br 2008;90(6):814–20.
35. Karpie JC, Chu CR. Lidocaine exhibits dose- and time-dependent cytotoxic effects on bovine articular chondrocytes in vitro. Am J Sports Med 2007;35(10):1621–7.

Soft Tissue Pathology of the Ankle

Benjamin D. Cullen, DPM, Glenn M. Weinraub, DPM*

KEYWORDS

• Soft • Tissue • Pathology • Ankle

Derangements of the soft tissues within the ankle joint can be secondary to a wide variety of pathophysiology. They typically involve synovial or fibrocartilaginous tissue and are chronic in nature.[1] Patients commonly present with persistent pain, swelling, and limitations on function. Left untreated, many of these conditions can progress to permanent joint degeneration. Fortunately, once diagnosed, they often respond well to current treatment options, with arthroscopic debridement playing a large role.

Suspicion for the presence of ankle soft tissue pathology is important to identifying it, as these disorders frequently have insidious onset and nonspecific symptoms. Evaluation should be guided by a detailed history and physical examination, followed by clinical, laboratory, and imaging studies as indicated. Although most symptoms are typically in the anterior compartment, the posterior ankle should also be examined, as pain sometimes may not be present with range of motion but will be elicited with palpation.

The etiology of ankle soft tissue disorders can be classified as traumatic injury, rheumatic disease, or congenital lesions. The pathophysiology, diagnosis, and management of these will be the focus of this article.

TRAUMATIC

Approximately 1 million acute ankle injuries occur annually in the United States, with the vast majority of these being diagnosed as lateral ankle sprains.[2] Depending on the severity of the trauma and the response of the tissue, sequelae can range from minimal and temporary inflammation to prolonged disability. As many as 15% to 20% of injuries can result in chronic symptoms.[3] For patients who have an extended recovery, common soft-tissue pathology includes nonspecific synovitis and secondary impingement lesions.

The authors have nothing to disclose.
Department of Orthopedic Surgery, Kaiser Hayward/Fremont, PMS-36, Rancho-Ohlone Building, 39400 Paseo Padre Parkway, Fremont, CA 94538, USA
* Corresponding author.
E-mail address: Glenn.m.Weinraub@kp.org

Clin Podiatr Med Surg 28 (2011) 469–480
doi:10.1016/j.cpm.2011.04.003
0891-8422/11/$ – see front matter © 2011 Elsevier Inc. All rights reserved.

Synovitis

The interior of the ankle capsule is lined by a synovial membrane, a tissue that functions to provide cushioning and lubrication for the joint. Often during an inversion sprain to the lateral collateral ligaments, some damage will occur to the synovium as well. This injury will result in irritation and inflammation, causing pain and swelling of the membrane. Symptoms can be local or generalized, but are typically limited to the anterolateral aspect of the joint.[4] Many times the sensation is vague, and discomfort only occurs with increases in activities.

On examination, patients with simple nonspecific synovitis will usually have minimal objective swelling and full range of motion. Radiographs will be negative, and unless there is a systemic component (eg, rheumatoid arthritis), laboratory work-up should be nonrevealing as well. Depending on the extent of tissue involved, there may be an altered signal intensity on magnetic resonance imaging (MRI), but often this can be equivocal. Of particular diagnostic value is injection of intra-articular anesthetic, which should provide significant relief. If not, then isolated synovitis is highly unlikely.

Initial treatment is conservative, with immobilization, physical therapy, nonsteroidal anti-inflammatory medication, and potentially corticosteroid injection, reserving surgery for resistant cases. If symptoms are refractory to these measures, arthroscopic debridement is the next step. Fortunately, nonspecific synovitis typically responds very well to this modality, and recovery time is minimal (**Figs. 1** and **2**). Radical excision is not necessary, as successful outcomes can be achieved with focus aimed specifically at pathologic tissue. Ferkel and colleagues[5] performed limited synovectomies on 31 patients, with 26 reporting good or excellent results. A postoperative regimen of physical therapy may be considered to limit swelling and enhance return of function, and overall the prognosis is good for these patients.

Impingement

Conditions that cause painful restriction of movement in the ankle joint due to tissue overgrowth are termed impingement syndromes (**Fig. 3**). In those cases where the limitation of motion is due to soft tissue hypertrophy, several distinct phenomena can be the cause. While the presence of impinging abnormal fibrous tissue in various forms and locations within the ankle joint has been thoroughly reported in the literature, the pathophysiology and certain characteristics of these lesions are subject to debate. However, the general consensus is that antecedent trauma of varying severity

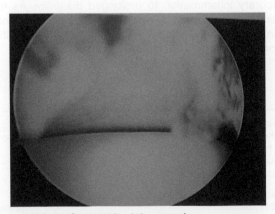

Fig. 1. Nonspecific synovitis to the anterior joint margin.

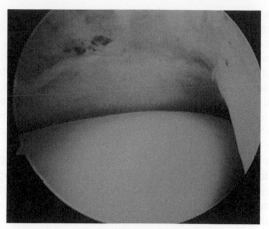

Fig. 2. The synovitis has been resected with a synovial shaver.

is typically associated with their development, usually in the form of a lateral ligament sprain.[6]

Wolin lesion
A mass of hyalinized connective tissue arising from the anteroinferior portion of the ankle joint was first described by Wolin and colleagues[7] in 1950. In their study of 9 patients with chronic anterolateral ankle joint pain and swelling following inversion injuries, a dense mass of white, fibrocartilaginous tissue was noted in the interval between the talus and the fibula upon arthrotomy. Wolin suggested the lesion developed as a result of incomplete resorption of post-traumatic tissue, wherein shear

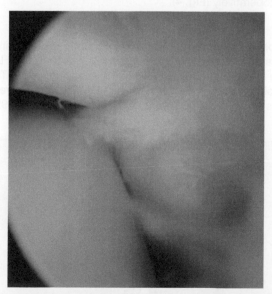

Fig. 3. Intraoperative view of anterolateral soft tissue impingement. The joint is a negative-pressure environment; thus one can see how this soft tissue would be impinged between the joint surfaces with normal dorsiflexion of the ankle.

forces between the talus and the fibula molded the scar tissue under pressure into an organized mass. As the presentation of the lesion was similar to that of a meniscus, he labeled it a meniscoid.

Controversy exists in terms of the nomenclature, as different authors have labeled similarly described pathology alternatively as plica syndrome,[8] fibrous bands,[9] or synovial impingement lesions.[10] It is likely that each of these exists on a continuum, with the organized meniscoid lesion being the well-differentiated end product. The nature of the scar tissue in question is also unclear, as traumatic synovitis was postulated by Wolin, whereas other authors endorsed a tear of the anterior talofibular ligament.[11]

Clinically, these lesions present as chronic post-traumatic pain and swelling, vaguely localized to the area of the anterolateral ankle joint. Although many patients complain of sensations of instability, objective findings are usually negative. Tenderness should be maximal along the anterolateral joint line or with compression of the fibula on the talus; however, these lesions can be intermittently asymptomatic. A potential finding is clicking or popping with ankle range of motion, which may or may not be painful.

The diagnosis is mostly based on history and physical examination, but imaging can be helpful in ruling out other pathology. Radiographs may show evidence of a previous inversion injury.

Computed tomography (CT) with contrast or MRI may reveal the presence of some abnormal soft tissue, but the potential for limited additional diagnostic value must be weighed against the cost of performing the test. As with other intra-articular soft tissue pathology, injection of anesthetic can be both therapeutic and diagnostic.

A trial of conservative therapy is not unwarranted with this condition; however, if a true organized meniscoid lesion is present, this is unlikely to be successful in eliminating symptoms. Fortunately, in all reported cases wherein an isolated mass of scar tissue was excised from the anterolateral gutter, patients have experienced significant improvement postoperatively (**Fig. 4**).

Bassett lesion

A lesion that is close in proximity to the meniscoid but a distinct clinical entity is the pathologic accessory anterior inferior tibiofibular ligament (AITFL). Bassett and colleagues[12] were the first to report an accessory fascicle of the AITFL as the cause of ligamentous impingement in the anterior ankle joint. An anatomic variant, the accessory fascicle, has been identified in anywhere from 21% to 92% of patients

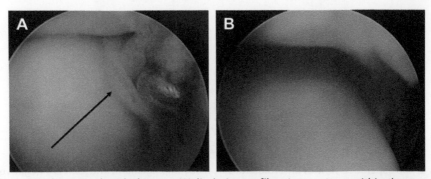

Fig. 4. (*A*) The arrow is pointing to a Wolin lesion or fibrotic scar tissue within the anterolateral ankle joint. (*B*) The subsequent picture shows the joint with the lesion debrided.

(depending on criteria) as a band oriented in parallel to the main ligament but separated from it by a fibrofatty septum.[13] The presence of this structure can therefore be considered a normal finding.

This accessory ligament can become pathologic following an inversion ankle injury that involves damage to the AITFL. If subsequent anterolateral hyperlaxity develops that results in anterior extrusion of the talar dome with dorsiflexion, the inferior fascicle of the AITFL will contact the talus with increased pressure and friction. This can often be reflected by the presence of an abraded area of the cartilage of the talus observed during arthroscopy. Bassett' lesion is thus a problem of abnormal positioning of normal anatomy (**Figs. 5** and **6**).

Much like Wolin lesion, the diagnosis of Bassett lesion should be considered in patients who have chronic ankle pain in the anterolateral region of the ankle after an inversion injury and have a stable ankle and normal plain radiographs. The main clinical difference between the 2 conditions will be the location of point tenderness, where in the case of Bassett lesion should be the anterolateral aspect of the talar dome and in the AITFL. Also, an audible popping and aggravation of pain with dorsiflexion and eversion have been reported to be more common with Bassett lesion than with other impingement lesions.[12]

Conservative management may be futile for this condition, as Akseki and colleagues[14] demonstrated that a regimen of physical therapy, nonsteroidal anti-inflammatory drugs (NSAIDs), and bracing for 3 months failed in all 21 patients they studied. In comparison, resection of the thickened and pathologic ligament was successful in relieving pain in these same patients (as well as those in Bassett's study), without causing any additional instability of the joint. A point to consider is that patients with less than 2 years of ankle pain before surgery for anterior ankle impingement showed significantly better scores in pain, swelling, ability to work, and engagement in sports postoperatively,[15] so prompt diagnosis and excision are key to better outcomes.

RHEUMATIC

Whereas post-traumatic lesions typically present as localized pain to the anterior aspect of the ankle joint, soft tissue disorders that have inflammatory (or unknown)

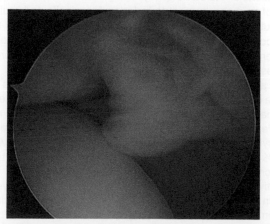

Fig. 5. A thickened inferior fascicle of the anterior inferior tibiofibular ligament that is impinging upon the lateral talar surface; this is subsequently resected.

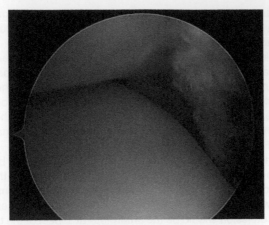

Fig. 6. The lesion in Fig. 5 following resection.

etiology can be symptomatic at virtually any anatomic site in this region. The diagnosis of these conditions is often more difficult, as onset is typically insidious with nonspecific clinical findings. Advanced imaging plays an enhanced role in investigation of these disorders, and frequently the process will only be definitively identified through histologic confirmation. Treatment is also less straightforward, as these lesions have a tendency for recurrence.

Pigmented Villonodular Synovitis

Pigmented villonodular synovitis (PVNS) is a relatively uncommon disorder characterized by proliferation of synovium, resulting in villous or nodular changes to synovial-lined joints, bursae, and tendon sheaths. The incidence has been reported as occurring in 1.8 patients per 1 million population annually, typically between the 2nd and 5th decades of life.[16] Both diffuse and local forms have been described based on the extent of tissue involvement, and Jaffe is credited with recognizing them as different presentations of the same entity.[17]

The presence of lipid and hemosiderin-laden foam cells and multinucleated giant cells has been routinely described on histologic analysis of lesions of PVNS, but the pathogenesis is controversial. Various mechanisms have been proposed, including localized lipid derangement, repeated nontraumatic inflammation, and a benign neoplastic process, but no definitive causality has been confirmed.

Due to its rarity and the nonspecific nature of symptoms, PVNS is often discovered incidentally or as a diagnosis of exclusion. It should be included in the differential diagnosis when monoarticular inflammation with or without a palpable mass presents in young patients. Persistent and generalized swelling, aching, and pain aggravated by activity are the symptoms typically expressed in the literature. Myers and Masi[16] reported that 53% of the 166 cases they studied had a history of trauma, but many case studies describe insidious onset without any inciting event.

Depending on the form and stage of PVNS, radiographs may reveal anything from subtle increases in soft tissue density to frank erosions of periarticular bone and subchondral cysts similar to that found in degenerative joint disease. A distinguishing characteristic between the 2 conditions is that PVNS is not associated with osteophyte formation.[18] MRI is very useful in diagnosis, as it reveals the presence of hemosiderin deposits, lipids, and inflammatory tissue, as well as the degree of invasion of cartilage or bone. The clinician should expect a low-signal intensity in the area of lesions on both T1- and T2-weighted images.[19] Aspiration of fluid that features brownish discoloration (due to hemosiderin) further reinforces the diagnosis.[20]

Conservative management is not indicated with a diagnosis of PVNS, as delay in definitive treatment could result in significant cartilage and bony destruction. Nodular lesions confined to a local area within the joint may respond well to simple excision, and have a lower reported incidence of recurrence.[21] With the diffuse form, complete synovectomy has been advocated as the treatment of choice, and some authors promote the concomitant use of hydrogen peroxide irrigation.[22] Long-term follow-up is essential in these patients, and the return of pathologic tissue following excision is usually treated with radiation therapy, often with good results.[23]

Synovial Chondromatosis

A rare disorder featuring multiple cartilaginous nodules originating within the synovium, primary synovial chondromatosis is a benign process, typically monoarticular, with symptomatic presentation reported most often between the 3rd and 5th decades of life (**Figs. 7** and **8**).[24] The exact pathophysiology is unclear, but leading theories suggest metaplasia of synovium into cartilaginous tissue versus a primary benign neoplasm. This is in contrast to secondary synovial chondromatosis, where arthritic conditions are the source of the pathologic tissue.

In 1977, Milgram classified synovial chondromatosis into 3 distinct phases.[25] Phase 1 features purely intrasynovial involvement. Active synovitis and nodule formation is present, but no loose bodies can be identified. Phase 2 is considered a transitional period. Nodular synovitis and now loose bodies are present in the joint, but these are primarily still cartilaginous. They may present similar to rice bodies seen in other inflammatory arthritides. In phase 3, the synovitis is quiescent, and the loose bodies are mostly calcified.

There was minimal difference in the duration of symptoms for patients in each of the 3 phases in Milgram's paper, and so the rate of progression from stage to stage likely varies considerably. In comparison, the quality of symptoms for each group was

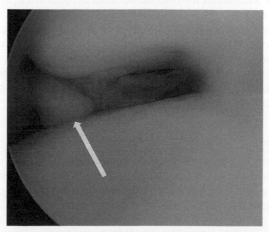

Fig. 7. Arthroscopic view of typical cartilaginous lesion seen with synovial chondromatosis. While this view is of 1 isolated lesion, it should be noted that a multitude of these loose bodies can be encountered within the joint.

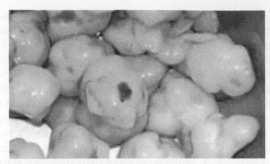

Fig. 8. Multiple loose bodies removed from a single joint with synovial chondromatosis.

significantly dissimilar. Patients with purely intrasynovial disease reported minimal pain, clicking, or locking; rather chronic swelling was their chief complaint. Those patients with phase 3 disease largely related pain and loss of motion. Patients in the transitional phase had a combination of symptoms from the other 2 phases.

Symptoms in all patients typically develop insidiously over a period of months to years.[26] Clinical findings at any stage may include crepitus, locking, pain, or limitation on range of motion, focal swelling, or palpable nodules. Plain films have greatest diagnostic value in phase 3 and late phase 2 disease when lesions have begun to calcify, with the presence of multiple intra-articular bodies of similar size and shape being very suggestive of the diagnosis.[27] CT and MRI can be very helpful in identifying and localizing lesions, although appearance will vary dramatically depending on the amount of calcification and synovial proliferation. Histologic examination confirms the diagnosis, and allows distinction between primary and secondary processes.

No formal recommendations for treatment exist, but the general consensus is that indications for surgery correlate with the phase of the disease. In phase 3, simple removal of the loose bodies has been shown to provide symptomatic relief with minimal complications.[28] However, when synovitis is present, failure to excise this pathologic tissue is associated with increased rates of recurrence, and so partial synovectomy is necessary.

As nodules have been observed to absorb over time and surgery predisposes patients to joint scarring, invasive procedures may be relatively contraindicated in asymptomatic patients.[29]

However, a relative risk of 5% of cases for malignant degeneration to chondrosarcoma has been reported,[30] so histologic diagnosis is prudent in all cases, especially for episodes of recurrence.

Crystalline Deposition

Derangements in the metabolism of monosodium urate (MSU) in gout and calcium pyrophosphate dihydrate (CPPD) in pseudogout can result in crystal deposition at any of various sites, including the ankle. Whereas MSU crystals precipitate in tissues systemically throughout the body as a result of purine catabolism, CPPD crystals are thought to be a primary disorder of articular cartilage associated with the production of inorganic pyrophosphate by chondrocytes.[31] With an identical macroscopic appearance and clinical presentation, distinction between the 2 processes can only be made with microscopic analysis.

Diagnosis of a crystalline deposition disease is fairly straightforward, as the differential of an acutely red, hot, swollen and excruciatingly painful joint is limited to few entities. The significance of the correlation between prolonged crystal deposition and the development and progression of osteoarthritis is less apparent. A strong association exists between the presence of crystals and cartilage degeneration,[32] but whether crystals preferentially deposit in damaged cartilage or if the changes they produce with chronic disease mimic that of osteoarthritis is unclear. The acute flares are considered to be caused by leukocyte ingestion of crystals, thus triggering an inflammatory cascade and extensive joint synovitis. Traditionally, cartilage wear was thought to result from repeated bouts of inflammation, but studies have shown that crystals can be present in uninflamed joints,[33] and so they may induce damage biomechanically.

Management of both diseases is currently primarily pharmacologic. Acute flare-ups can be treated with colchicine, NSAIDs, and potentially injected or oral corticosteroids. Elevated serum uric acid may be controlled with indefinite use of daily medications. If these conservative measures fail to alleviate inflammation, arthroscopic lavage has been advocated as a secondary option for acute attacks (**Fig. 9**).[1] Removal of crystals in asymptomatic joints may prevent future flares, but this has not been thoroughly reported on. If gouty tophi provide discomfort or affect function, these may potentially be excised, but this should be accompanied by medical therapy to limit hyperuricemia and the recurrence of lesions.

Rheumatoid Arthritis

A thorough discussion of the pathophysiology and treatment of rheumatoid arthritis (RA) is beyond the scope of this article. This disorder of the immune system characterized by global synovial hyperplasia and inflammatory cell proliferation is mentioned here as another instance (besides diffuse PVNS) in which aggressive synovectomy may be indicated. As opposed to the majority of pathology described elsewhere in this article in which a limited surgical approach is sufficient, RA features widespread involvement of the synovium. If debridement is to be performed, most authors who advocate it suggest near total excision for maximum benefit and to limit recurrence of symptoms. Beyond providing excellent access to the inflamed tissue, an open arthrotomy will also allow any necessary tenosynovectomy to be accomplished simultaneously. Although the procedure is controversial, it is an option for patients with disease that is inadequately controlled by conservative measures.

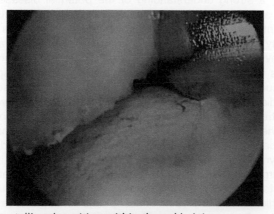

Fig. 9. Advanced crystalline deposition within the ankle joint.

CONGENITAL

Plicae are natural folds of synovial tissue that are found in the anterior, posterior, or syndesmotic recesses of the ankle joint.[34] These loose, pliable, and elastic projections normally move freely on the articular surface with joint motion. Plica syndrome refers to the painful impairment of joint function in which the only finding that helps explain the symptoms is the presence of a thickened and fibrotic plica. It is unclear what causes plicae to become symptomatic; however, overuse and trauma have been suggested etiologies.

Unless pathologic, plicae are not usually associated with local reactive signs. The primary symptom of plica syndrome is pain; however, there may also be a snapping sensation within the joint as the thickened plica is rubbed by bony structures during range of motion. Sometimes a band of tissue is palpable, and if the plica becomes severely irritated, joint swelling may occur. Plicae can be differentiated from meniscoid lesions in that they are not seen in the talofibular interval.[34]

Identification of plica syndrome is primarily through exclusion of other causes for symptoms. Radiographs, CT, and MRI may be used to rule out coexisting pathology, but are often unnecessary. If the history and physical strongly suggest the presence of a symptomatic plica, and conservative measures fail to provide adequate relief, arthroscopy may be indicated for both diagnostic and therapeutic purposes. Resection is curative, and no known sequelae are associated with the removal of plicae.

SUMMARY

The spectrum of pathology that can involve the intra-articular soft tissues of the ankle joint ranges from acute and self-limited to chronic and debilitating. While some form of trauma is implicated in the development of many of these conditions, the exact pathophysiology is still largely theoretical at this time. This is especially evident when comparing patients with the same disorder, yet with dramatically different accounts of the severity of any associated injury. Confounding matters even further is the wide variation in nature and progression of symptoms for the same process in different patients. Clearly, although a single inciting episode may initiate the cascade of events, host susceptibility is also very important to how the disease develops.

Diagnosis should be pursued through an algorithmic approach. A detailed history and physical examination are usually the most critical aspects of the work-up, followed closely by a strong understanding of the potential disease processes that can occur at this anatomic location. The value of a diagnostic injection of anesthetic for determining intra-articular pathology cannot be overstated, as this is a simple and easy modality with high yield. Imaging studies such as radiograph, CT and MRI can be useful in evaluating the presence and extent of a particular condition, or ruling out other causes for symptoms. If the clinician has a strong suspicion that intra-articular soft tissue pathology is present, proceeding with arthroscopy of the joint can confirm the diagnosis while simultaneously allowing for definitive treatment.

The nature of treatment pathways for these disorders depends on the severity of symptoms and the natural course of the disease. Conservative management such as activity modification, NSAIDs, physical therapy, and corticosteroid use may be indicated with mild symptoms or a process that will not eventually result in deterioration of the joint. More urgency is associated with a condition that is disabling or that can cause permanent arthrosis. In those instances, surgical correction may have to be pursued at an earlier interval to prevent unacceptable consequences that would result from delay in action. Fortunately, most of the derangements presented here respond very well to debridement, and overall the prognosis is very good for this category of pathology.

REFERENCES

1. Guhl JF, Boynton MD. Soft tissue pathology. In: Guhl JF, Parisien JS, Boynton MD, editors. Arthroscopy of the foot and ankle. 3rd edition. New York: Springer-Verlag; 2004. p. 99–114.
2. Wexler RK. The injured ankle. Am Fam Physician 1998;57(3):474–80.
3. Ogilvie-Harris DJ, Gilbart MK, Chorney K. Chronic pain following ankle sprains in athletes the role of arthroscopic surgery. Arthroscopy 1997;13:564–74.
4. Meislin RJ, Rose DJ, Parisien JS, et al. Arthroscopic treatment of synovial impingement of the ankle. Am J Sports Med 1993;21:186–9.
5. Ferkel RD, Karzel RP, Del Pizzo W, et al. Arthroscopic treatment of anterolateral impingement of the ankle. Am J Sports Med 1991;19(5):440–6.
6. Umans H. Ankle impingement syndromes. Semin Musculoskelet Radiol 2002;6: 133–9.
7. Wolin I, Glassman F, Sideman S, et al. Internal derangement of the talofibular component of the ankle. Surg Gynecol Obstet 1950;91:193–200.
8. Gächter A, Gerber BE. Arthroskopie des oberen Sprunggelenkes in Lokalanäs-thesie [arthroscopy of the ankle under local anesthesia]. Arthroskopie 1991;4: 37–41 [in German].
9. Schonholtz GJ. Arthoscopic surgery of the ankle joint. Arthoscopic surgery of the shoulder, elbow, and ankle. Springfield (IL): Charles C Thomas; 1986. p. 59–72.
10. Stone JW, Guhl JF. Meniscoid lesions of the ankle. Clin Sports Med 1991;10: 661–76.
11. Andrews JR, Drez DJ, McGinty JB. Symposium: arthroscopy of joints other than the knee. Contemp Orthop 1984;9:71–100.
12. Bassett FH III, Gates HS III, Billys JB, et al. Talar impingement by the anteroinfe-rior tibiofibular ligament. J Bone Joint Surg Am 1990;72:55–9.
13. Nikolopoulos CE, Tsirikos AI, Sourmelis S, et al. The accessory anteroinferior tibiofibular ligament as a cause of talar impingement: a cadaveric study. Am J Sports Med 2004;32:389–95.
14. Akseki D, Pinar H, Bozkurt M, et al. The distal fascicle of the anterior inferior tibio-fibular ligament as a cause of anterolateral ankle impingement. Acta Orthop Scand 1999;70(5):478–82.
15. van Dijk CN, Tol JL, Verheyen CC. A prospective study of prognostic factors con-cerning the outcome of arthroscopic surgery for anterior ankle impingement. Am J Sports Med 1997;26(6):737–45.
16. Myers BW, Masi AT. Pigmented villonodular synovitis and tenosynovitis: a clinical epidemiologic study of 166 cases and literature review. Medicine 1980;59:223–38.
17. Jaffe HL, Lichtenstein L, Sutro CJ. Pigmented villonodular synovitis, bursitis and tenosynovitis. Arch Pathol 1941;31:731–65.
18. Smith JH, Pugh DG. Roentgenographic aspects of articular pigmented villonod-ular synovitis. Am J Roentgenol Radium Ther Nucl Med 1962;87:1146–56.
19. Mandelbaum BR, Grant TT, Hartzman S, et al. The use of MRI to assist in diag-nosis of pigmented villonodular synovitis of the knee joint. Clin Orthop 1988; 231:135–9.
20. Rao AS, Vigorita VJ. Pigmented villonodular synovitis (giant cell tumor of the tendon sheath and synovial membrane). A review of 81 cases. J Bone Joint Surg Am 1984;66:76–94.

21. Flandry F, Hughston JC. Pigmented villonodular synovitis. J Bone Joint Surg Am 1987;69:942–9.

22. Saxena A, Perez H. Pigmented villonodular synovitis about the ankle: a review of the literature and presentation in 10 athletic patients. Foot Ankle Int 2004;25: 819–26.

23. O'Sullivan B, Cummings B, Catton C, et al. Outcome following radiation treatment for high-risk pigmented villonodular synovitis. Int J Radiat Oncol Biol Phys 1995; 32:777–86.

24. Iossifidis A, Sutaria PD, Pinto T. Synovial chondromatosis of the ankle. Foot 1995; 5:44–6.

25. Milgram JW. Synovial osteochondromatosis: a histopathological study of thirty cases. J Bone Joint Surg Am 1977;59:792–801.

26. Krebbs VE. The role of hip arthroscopy in the treatment of synovial disorders and loose bodies. Clin Orthop Relat Res 2003;406:48–59.

27. Murphey MD, Vidal JA, Fanburg-Smith JC, et al. Imaging of synovial chondromatosis with radiologic–pathologic correlation. Radiographics 2007;27:1465–88.

28. Young-in Lee F, Hornicek FJ, Dick HM, et al. Synovial chondromatosis of the foot. Clin Orthop Relat Res 2004;423:186–90.

29. Yu GV, Zema RL, Johnson RW. Synovial osteochondromatosis. A case report and review of the literature. J Am Podiatr Med Assoc 2002;92:247–54.

30. Davis RI, Hamilton A, Biggart JD. Primary synovial chondromatosis: a clinicopathologic review and assessment of malignant potential. Hum Pathol 1998;29(7): 683–8.

31. Silcox DC, McCarty DJ. Elevated inorganic pyrophosphate concentration in synovial fluid in osteoarthritis and pseudogout. J Lab Clin Med 1974;83:518–31.

32. Hayes A, Harris B, Dieppe P, et al. Wear of articular cartilage: the effect of crystals. Proc Inst Mech Eng 1993;207:41–58.

33. Martinez-Sanchez A, Pascual E. Intracellular and extracellular CPPD crystals are a regular feature in synovial fluid from uninflamed joints of patients with CPPD related arthropathy. Ann Rheum Dis 2005;64:1769–72.

34. Stienstra JJ. Intra-articular soft-tissue masses of the ankle. Meniscoid lesions and transarticular fibrous bands. Clin Podiatr Med Surg 1994;11(3):371–83.

Arthroscopic Treatment of Ankle Osteochondral Lesions

Tanya J. Singleton, DPM[a], Byron Hutchinson, DPM[b],
Lawrence Ford, DPM[c],*

KEYWORDS

• Osteochondral lesion • Talar dome lesion • Ankle
• Arthroscopy

Osteochondral lesions (OCLs) of the ankle represent a host of pathologies, from subtle chondromalacia to full-thickness defects with underlying cystic changes and osteonecrosis. Frequently these lesions are traumatic in origin, most commonly occurring after an acute ankle sprain; however, atraumatic mechanisms have been described. Osteochondral lesions of the talus (OLT) are more common than lesions of the tibial plafond. In their landmark paper, Berndt and Harty[1] delineated both a classification system and a clarification of the behavior of these injuries, focusing on mechanism and location of the lesion.

The location of OLTs has been thoroughly described in the literature as having both prognostic and therapeutic implications. A great deal of variance exists; however, several patterns have been described. Medial lesions tend to be more common and, although often atraumatic in origin, can occur from inversion and plantar flexion ankle injuries. Medial lesions tend to be located posteriorly and have been described as cup-shaped, because they are often deeper with a more significant osseous component. Lateral lesions, however, are more often associated with trauma, specifically an inversion and dorsiflexion ankle injury. Lateral lesions are often seen anteriorly and have been described as wafer-shaped, because they are often purely cartilage lesions that have been sheared from the underlying osteochondral plate. This finding

The authors have nothing to disclose.
[a] Kaiser San Francisco Bay Area Foot and Ankle Residency Program, 280 West MacArthur Boulevard, Oakland, CA 94611, USA
[b] Franciscan Medical Group, International Foot & Ankle Foundation, Franciscan Foot & Ankle Institute, Highline, 16233 Sylvester Road South West G-10, Seattle, WA 98166, USA
[c] Kaiser San Francisco Bay Area Foot and Ankle Residency Program, Department of Orthopedics and Podiatric Surgery, Kaiser Permanente, 280 West MacArthur Boulevard, Oakland, CA 94611, USA
* Corresponding author.
E-mail address: Lawrence.Ford@kp.org

Clin Podiatr Med Surg 28 (2011) 481–490
doi:10.1016/j.cpm.2011.04.006
0891-8422/11/$ – see front matter © 2011 Elsevier Inc. All rights reserved.

is not a consistent rule, because OLTs can have variable appearance throughout the talar dome. Theoretically, medial lesions with their larger osseous component have a better chance of consolidating with the underlying bone and its blood supply with proper treatment, which may range from immobilization to microfracture or open reduction and internal fixation. Lateral lesions lack this inherent advantage and may have less-predictable outcomes.

Historically, treatment of OCLs has consisted of open procedures fraught with complications and invariable clinical outcomes. Open procedures often require malleolar osteotomies and use of autologous harvest, often from the knee or allograft. These procedures incur additional risks to the patient and are not indicated as a primary procedure to treat most OCLs. Arthroscopic treatment of ankle OCLs has the advantage of a minimally invasive approach, allowing for thorough evaluation of pathology and multiple treatment modalities.

PATHOPHYSIOLOGY

The pathophysiology of OCLs must be appreciated to fully understand why the various treatment modalities are effective and when to use them. The initial insult involves some level of joint or articular damage, whether from trauma or other metabolic, genetic, vascular, or idiopathic processes.[2] Many lesions are often traced back to a specific ankle sprain, ankle fracture, or other lower extremity trauma.[3] Alternatively, nonspecific repetitive microtrauma may generate an OCL over time, or asymptomatic necrotic lesions may become symptomatic with subtle injuries. Regardless of the inciting event or baseline pathology, the processes through which these lesions become symptomatic are the same. Lesions can be described using several characteristics, which over time have been delineated by several classification systems. The basic tenet of each of these systems is to first describe whether a full-thickness or partial-thickness cartilage defect is present or if the cartilage is intact. The quality and condition of the subchondral bone plate and the underlying trabecular bone are important to know. A fragment of bone may be attached to the disrupted cartilage. The subchondral plate may be fractured or compacted and the underlying bone may have become sclerotic. Subchondral cyst formation may have occurred. These features should be noted and may offer clues as to the physiologic process and appropriate treatment (**Fig. 1**). Whether the fragment is partially or fully detached or displaced should also be noted. Understanding these dynamics of the lesion provides clues to the origin and may assist in directing treatment.

Partial-thickness or full-thickness flaps of cartilage that have separated from the underlying subchondral bone are created through shearing forces and are not amenable to being left alone to repair themselves because of lack of blood supply. They will act as an irritant in the joint space, promoting synovial inflammation and subsequent symptoms. Sometimes this synovitis is more symptomatic to the patient than the lesion itself. These cartilage flaps have been recently called *chondral-separated lesions*, in contradistinction to osteochondral-separated lesions.[4] This latter type of lesion is more commonly referred to as an osteochondral fracture and may have a better chance of forming fibrocartilage because of its retained blood supply from the subchondral bone.

Cysts may form with either chondral or osteochondral lesions when the subchondral plate is compromised. Where small defects in the subchondral plate exist, repetitive loading from normal weight-bearing activates forces the synovial fluid under high pressure into the subchondral bone, which over time creates a cyst.[5,6] Cystic lesions may also be seen with apparently intact cartilage. This finding can be explained by a similar

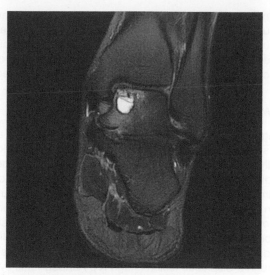

Fig. 1. T2-weighted coronal image of an osteochondral lesion of the talus with subchondral cyst formation. Extravasation of synovial fluid through the compromised cartilage is believed to cause instability in the underlying bony substrate.

mechanism in which the subchondral plate is fractured and the fluid content of the cartilage is exsanguinated and forced into the subchondral bone with repetitive weight-bearing pressures. As the cyst develops and the integrity of the subchondral plate collapses, the overlying cartilage becomes soft because of the absence of this supportive structure. Over time, as these cavities are continually filled with fluid under pressure, the bone reabsorbs, creating a subchondral cyst, which may become sclerotic as the exposed bone remodels.[5,6] Whether these lesions are caused by trauma or local necrosis, they may evolve to include sclerotic areas of bone with associated subchondral cyst formation. The theory of these nuances led to the development of many of the operative treatments currently used. Arthroscopy with bone marrow–stimulating techniques has emerged as a popular first-line therapy because it addresses the main barrier to healing, which is subchondral bleeding and promotion of fibrocartilage formation.

A basic knowledge of cartilage anatomy and physiology helps in understanding of the goals, mechanism, and limitations of arthroscopic treatment of OCLs. Native articular cartilage consists of hyaline cartilage. Hyaline cartilage is unique in that its matrix consists of primarily type II collagen, which has improved tensile strength over type I collagen, the predominant component of fibrocartilage. Hyaline cartilage, however, cannot be regenerated once injured. Fibrocartilage is the natural repair and physiologic alternative. Hyaline cartilage has abundant water content, accounting for approximately 75% of the cartilage matrix.[5,6] The matrix also contains fillers such as proteoglycans that aid in resisting compressive forces. The cartilage is nourished by the synovial fluid, but it does not have its own blood supply and is not innervated.[5,6] Articular cartilage can be divided into four zones.[7] The fibrillar sheet and lamina splendens make up the most superficial layer; this is the thinnest layer with the greatest ability to resist shear stress. Once violated, degradation and fibrillation become progressive, manifesting as a combination of any of the lesions previously described, depending on local physiology and external stress. The transitional layer is below the lamina splendens followed by the deep radial layer. The deep radial layer is the largest layer distributing force and resisting compression. The deepest layer is the calcified cartilage, the beginning of which is called the tidemark, which separates the hyaline cartilage from the underlying subchondral bone. This layer is significant in osteochondral repair procedures involving allograft or autograft material, because the tidemark level differs between different areas of individual joints and different joints themselves, thus having significant implications on loading and healing characteristics.

DIAGNOSIS AND WORKUP

Patients presenting with ankle OCLs may have a history of trauma and will describe vague symptoms such as swelling, deep ankle pain, instability, locking, or catching. The pain is typically difficult to reproduce on examination but can be confirmed with a response to a diagnostic ankle block. Lesions may be identified on plain radiographs. Ancillary imaging studies are useful when a high clinical suspicion exists or further clarification of the extent and nature of the lesion is needed. These studies often assist in preoperative planning. Several imaging specific classification systems have been developed with this goal in mind. Bernt and Harty's[1] classification system is based on plain radiographs and includes four stages from compression of the cartilage (stage 1) through a displaced lesion (stage IV). Although this system is useful, it has little prognostic value and as many as 50% of OCLs are missed on plain radiographs, necessitating advanced imaging.[8]

CT, although it accurately assesses the extent of bone involvement, is unable to assess the extent of the chondral injury, which is important in preoperative planning. Ferkel and colleagues[9] developed a classification scheme based on CT describing the osseous component with respect to cystic changes and communication with the joint surface.

MRI has gained popularity in its ability to delineate both the cartilage and bone extent of the lesion in addition to associated soft tissue pathology. Several MRI classification systems have been proposed, most of which stage lesions from chondral bruising through a detached fragment with a focus on the quality of the cartilage and the nature or absence of its attachments.[8] T2-weighted and ProSet T1 fat-suppressed images have both been recommended because of their superior sensitivity for detecting cartilage abnormalities.[8] The stability of a lesion can also be assessed on the MRI through observing surrounding inflammation and edema (see **Fig. 1**), although this is of unknown importance for preoperative planning and prognosis.

On T2-weighted images, increased signal intensity can be seen surrounding completely detached lesions, and bone edema may be present. These findings have been considered evidence of instability, which has been used as an operative indication; however, no clear correlation exists. In their recent work exploring why only some osteochondral defects in the ankle are painful, van Dijk and colleagues[5] attribute painful lesions to the repetitive increased fluid pressures. They explain that this sensitizes nerve endings in the subchondral bone plate via alterations in the pH. MRI is the best imaging modality to detect evidence of high fluid pressures surrounding lesions, which manifest as high signal intensity around the lesion and bone marrow edema on fat-suppressed images. Therefore, if painful lesions are assumed to be painful because of instability, these MRI findings are consistent with both.

Plain radiographs, CT, and MRI are all intended to help with treatment selection and preoperative planning where indicated; however, MRI seems to offer the most useful information and should be performed in most cases. Surgeons are cautioned that MRI may exaggerate the extent of osseous involvement in OCLs.[8] A threshold beyond which arthroscopy is unlikely to yield satisfactory results has been shown to exist around lesions greater than 1.5 cm^2.[10–12]

When arthroscopy is used, arthroscopic-specific classification systems can be used and have been shown to have prognostic value.[13] Several arthroscopic staging systems have been introduced. Pritsch[14] introduced a three-stage system in 1986 describing the cartilage as intact, soft, or frayed. In 1995, Ferkel and colleagues[13] introduced a more elaborate system that included stages A through F, in which A through C describe worsening grades of cartilage wear and stages D through F describe progressive lifting, detachment, and displacement of the fragment (**Box 1**).

INDICATIONS AND CONTRAINDICATIONS

Obvious fragments, unstable lesions and painful lesions that have otherwise failed to respond to conservative therapy should be considered for arthroscopic treatment. Variable recommendations have been made in the literature regarding the duration of conservative treatment before surgical intervention, whether it is open or arthroscopic. Some authors advocate earlier intervention, because prolonged preoperative symptoms may correlate with worse outcomes. A period of 4 to 6 weeks of immobilization is often attempted before surgical intervention.[2,15] In general, children and adolescents are more amenable to conservative care, and therefore arthroscopic treatment is considered only after aggressive conservative treatment has failed. Arthroscopy is indicated for ankle OCLs as both a diagnostic and therapeutic modality. It is most successful as a primary procedure, with less-satisfactory outcomes in revision surgery. Lesions less than 1.5 cm^2 are more amenable to arthroscopic treatment than larger lesions.[10–12] Relative contraindications include infection and severe degenerative joint disease.

SURGICAL TECHNIQUE

Arthroscopic treatment of ankle OCLs can be performed using standard anteromedial and anterolateral ankle portals. Sometimes a third posterolateral portal can help in

---

Box 1
Ferkel and colleagues rating: arthroscopic surgical grade based on status of articular cartilage

Grade A

   Smooth and intact, but soft or ballotable

Grade B

   Rough surface

Grade C

   Fibrillations/fissures

Grade D

   Flap present or bone exposed

Grade E

   Loose, undisplaced fragment

Grade F

   Displaced fragment

Ferkel and colleagues,[13] 2008

visualization and treatment of posterior lesions. A tourniquet may be necessary if hemostasis is not optimal; alternatively, the inflow may be supplemented with epinephrine. Anatomic location of lesions should be considered for optimal instrumentation. When using standard anteromedial and anterolateral portals, the camera is best inserted from the portal opposite the lesion, and ancillary instrumentation from the ipsilateral portal. For posterior lesions that may be difficult to reach from anterior portals, a noninvasive ankle joint distracter can improve visualization and access. Either a 2.7- or 4.0-mm scope can be used depending on surgeon preference. Both 30° and 70° models are helpful for complete visualization of all surfaces of the ankle joint.

The stepwise approach to treatment begins with inspection of the joint. To fully appreciate the lesions, a thorough debridement of synovitis, bands, and loose bodies should be performed using arthroscopic shavers and graspers as appropriate. This process allows improved visualization of the cartilage surfaces of the ankle joint. Full appreciation of all articular damage is possible through both visual inspection and probing. Fibrillations and delaminated flaps of cartilage can also be differentiated using a blunt arthroscopic probe. Firm areas of cartilage suggest normal intact cartilage that is attached to the underlying subchondral bone. Soft areas of cartilage suggest that the attachment between the cartilage and the underlying subchondral bone is compromised. These areas indicate an unstable lesion and do not have the potential to heal. Areas where the cartilage is soft but appears intact likely indicate underlying cystic formation. Once the extent of the damage is appreciated a plan to repair the lesions can be developed.

Unstable or loose areas of cartilage should be sharply demarcated and excised with perpendicular edges (**Fig. 2**). The purpose of this is to provide a circumferential barrier to hold the fibrocartilage plug in place during the healing process (**Fig. 3**). The goal is to promote bleeding of the underlying trabecular bone beneath the subchondral bone plate to facilitate fibrocartilage formation.

Where the cartilage is soft and yet intact, drilling of the underlying subchondral cyst without excision of the overlying cartilage can be performed. Both anterograde and retrograde approaches have been described with arthroscopic assistance.[16,17] The anterograde approach is performed by drilling directly through the anterior portals using a soft tissue protector. This technique is useful for very anterior lesions. The transmalleolar approach can be accomplished with or without the Micro Vector Drill Guide System (Smith & Nephew, Andover, MA, USA) and is useful for more posterior

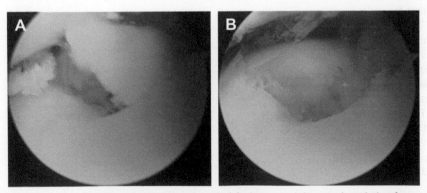

Fig. 2. (*A, B*) The borders of the osteochondral lesion are delineated and the fragment excised.

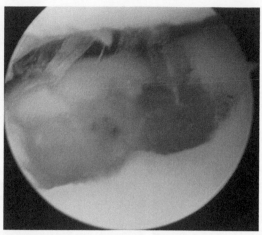

Fig. 3. Perpendicular walls are created before the subchondral bone is prepared for fibro-cartilage ingrowth.

lesions. The argument against these approaches is that intact cartilage is violated on the talus and the tibia in the transmalleolar approach. The retrograde transtalar approach may also be used when the cartilage is intact.[18] This approach not only allows for sufficient drilling of the subchondral bone and plate through a sinus tarsi approach but also allows the lesion to be backfilled. This process is accomplished by using a larger-gauge drill guide over the pin and introducing bone graft material through the tunnel after the pin is removed. During this technique, the intact cartilage of the talus is directly visualized via arthroscopy to ensure it is not violated during the drilling or packing procedures. When using nonarthroscopic power instrumentation as described, care should be taken to provide adequate irrigation at the level of the skin to prevent thermal injury.

When the cartilage is noted to be detached at any edge during the initial inspection, it must be sharply excised with clean perpendicular borders as described. Any underlying detached bone fragments or evidence of osteonecrosis must also be aggressively debrided to healthy bleeding bone. Excision of lesions without additional treatment of the underlying surface is not advocated. Once exposed, the subchondral bone can be prepared through drilling, abrasion, or microfracture techniques (**Fig. 4**). Drilling has already been described. Abrasion can be performed using curved curettes or an arthroscopic rotary burr.

The microfracture technique has gained popularity for its simplicity and excellent short- and medium-term outcomes.[10–12,19–21] This technique uses variable-angled awl instruments designed to penetrate the subchondral plate 3 to 4 mm. This technique requires penetrating the lesion with the awl in a centripetal fashion, starting treatment at the perimeter and working inward, spacing the insertion points approximately 2 to 3 mm apart so that the subchondral bridges do not break.

Each of these techniques is also meant to create a rough surface, which can attract and hold the marrow clot for the formation of healing fibrocartilage. These techniques are collectively referred to as *bone marrow stimulation*.

POSTOPERATIVE PROTOCOL

Immediate postoperative protocol consists of non–weight-bearing exercises until the skin heals and sutures are removed. Early range of motion is important; however, early

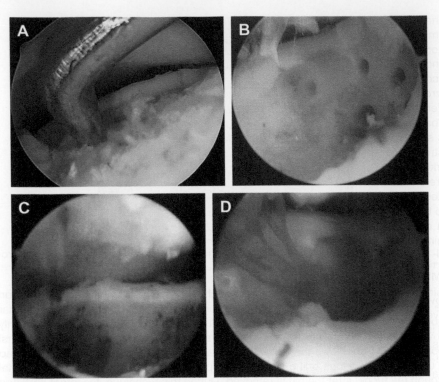

Fig. 4. Microfracture using a small awl (*A*), drilling with K-wires (*B*), or abrasion arthroplasty (*C*) are effective ways to facilitate bleeding from the underlying trabecular bone (*D*).

weight-bearing is controversial. The authors recommend early range of motion with continued non–weight-bearing activities for a full 4 to 6 weeks. This latter protocol is especially required for larger cystic lesions. Patients may take 12 to 18 weeks to experience significant symptom relief after arthroscopic treatment, although complete healing can take several months to a year.

OUTCOMES

Outcomes of arthroscopic treatment of ankle OCLs are generally good with a low complication profile. Larger lesions and increased duration of symptoms preoperatively tend to impact results negatively. In 2010, Lee and colleagues[21] published a statistically significant increase in American Orthopaedic Foot and Ankle Scores, with greater than 89% good to excellent results with arthroscopic microfracture of talus lesions less than 15 mm with average follow-up of 33 months. In their study, a negative correlation was found between duration of symptoms preoperatively and clinical outcomes, with a significant difference in outcomes noted for patients experiencing symptoms for more than 1 year compared with those experiencing symptoms for less than 1 year at the time of operative intervention. In an earlier study, Lee and colleagues[22] took a second look with arthroscopy and showed that lesions were incompletely repaired at 12 months postoperatively; however, clinical outcomes were good and consistent with the authors' most recent series. In 2008, Chuckpaiwong and colleagues[11] published results on 105 ankle OCLs treated with microfracture, showing 70% successful results. They found a strong correlation between the size of the lesion and successful outcomes, with deteriorating results in lesions larger than 15 mm. Qin-wei and colleagues[10] echoed this finding in their retrospective analysis, reporting poorer results in lesions larger than 10 mm. In 2009, Choi and colleagues[12] found that 150 mm^2 represented a critical defect size at and beyond which poorer outcomes were seen in their cohort of 120 ankles that underwent arthroscopic marrow–stimulating techniques for OCLs of the talus.

Ferkel and colleagues[13] published results on the arthroscopic treatment of 50 patients with OCLs of the talus, with an average of 71 months of follow-up. In this study, good to excellent outcomes were seen in 64% to 72% of patients, with a strong correlation noted between their expanded arthroscopic grading system (Ferkel and colleagues[13]) and clinical outcomes (see **Box 1**). They determined that more unstable lesions (D–F) responded worse than stable lesions (A–C). OCLs associated with soft tissue impingement, particularly anterior lateral ankle impingement, also tend to respond better, which may be because of the arthroscopic synovectomy that often accompanies the treatment of an OCL, highlighting the ambiguity of the origin of pain associated with these lesions.

COMPLICATIONS

A low complication rate is associated with arthroscopic treatment of ankle OCLs. Nerve injury manifesting as neuritis or portal pain is the most common complication and is typically self-limiting. A low incidence of superficial and deep wound complications is associated with this minimal incision approach. Continued pain and progression of symptoms can be seen. Where further surgical intervention is sought, the impact that the loss of the subchondral plate integrity from marrow-stimulating techniques will have on future surgical options is not well defined. Although marrow-stimulating techniques are widely regarded as non–bridge-burning procedures, this tenet may not be true for larger or more chronic lesions.[23]

SUMMARY

Arthroscopic treatment of OCLs of the ankle is a popular first-line surgical option after conservative therapy has failed. MRI is the preferred imaging modality to evaluate OCLs and aid in surgical planning. Associated soft tissue pathology must be appreciated and addressed surgically, because associated synovitis and soft tissue impingement often contribute to symptoms. The diverse treatment modalities available via arthroscopy offer simplistic and straightforward solutions for biologically and mechanically complicated pathology. Marrow-stimulating techniques, particularly microfracture, have shown good to excellent results in most patients with small (<15 mm) acute lesions, and have a low complication rate.

REFERENCES

1. Berndt AL, Harty M. Transchondral fractures (osteochondritis dissecans) of the talus. J Bone Joint Surg 1959;42(6):988–1020.
2. Grossman J, Lyons M. A review of osteochondral lesions of the talus. Clin Podiatr Med Surg 2009;26(2):205–26.
3. Aktas S, Kocaoglu B, Gereli A, et al. Incidence of chondral lesions of talar dome in ankle fracture types. Foot Ankle Int 2008;29(3):287–92.
4. Monden S, Hasegawa A, Takagishi K. A clinical study of chondral-separated types of osteochondral lesions of the talus. Foot Ankle Int 2010;31(2):124–30.

5. van Dijk CN, Reilingh ML, Zengerink M, et al. Osteochondral defects in the ankle: why painful? Knee Surg Sports Traumatol Arthrosc 2010;18:570–80.

6. Van Dijk CN, Reilingh ML, Zengerink M, et al. The natural history of osteochondral lesions in the ankle. Knee Surg Sports Traumatol Arthrosc 2010;59:375–86.

7. Martin RB, Burr DB, Sharkey NA. Skeletal tissue mechanics. New York: Springer-Verlag Inc; 1998. p. 50–5.

8. O'Loughlin PF, Heyworth BE, Kennedy JG. Current concepts in the diagnosis and treatment of osteochondral lesions of the ankle. Am J Sports Med 2010;38(2): 392–404.

9. Ferkel RD, Sgaglion NA, Del Pizzo W, et al. Arthroscopic treatment of osteochondral lesions of the talus: techniques and results. Ortho Trans 1990;14:272.

10. Qin-wei G, Yue-lin H, Chen J, et al. Arthroscopic treatment for osteochondral lesions of the talus: analysis of outcome predictors. Chin Med J 2010;123(3): 296–300.

11. Chuckpaiwong B, Berkson EM, Theodore GH. Microfracture for osteochondral lesions of the ankle: outcome analysis and outcome predictors of 105 cases. Arthroscopy 2008;24(1):106–12.

12. Choi WJ, Park KK, Kim BS, et al. Osteochondral lesion of the talus: is there a critical defect size for poor outcome? Am J Sports Med 2009;37(10):1974–80.

13. Ferkel RD, Zanotti RM, Komenda GA, et al. Arthroscopic treatment of chronic osteochondral lesions of the talus: long-term results. Am J Sports Med 2008; 36(90):1750–62.

14. Pritsch M, Horoshovski H, Farine I. Arthroscopic treatment of osteochondral lesions of the talus. J Bone Joint Surg Am 1986;68(6):862–5.

15. van Dijk C, Van Bergen C. Advancements in ankle arthroscopy. J Am Acad Orthop Surg 2008;16(11):635–46.

16. Easley M, Latt L, Santangelo J, et al. Osteochondral lesions of the talus. J Am Acad Orthop Surg 2010;18(10):616–30.

17. Zengerink M, Struijs PAA, Tol JL, et al. Treatment of osteochondral lesions of the talus: a systematic review. Knee Surg Sports Traumatol Arthrosc 2010;18:238–46.

18. Ferkel R, Scranton P, Kern B. Surgical treatment of osteochondral lesions of the talus. AAOS Instr Course Lec 2010;59:387–403.

19. McGahan PJ, Pinney SJ. Current concept review: osteochondral lesions of the talus. Foot Ankle Int 2010;31(1):90–101.

20. O'Driscoll SW. Current concepts review—the healing and regeneration of articular cartilage. J Bone Joint Surg Am 1998;80:1795–812.

21. Lee KB, Bai LB, Chung JY. Arthroscopic microfracture for osteochondral lesions of the talus. Knee Surg Sports Traumatol Arthrosc 2010;18:247–53.

22. Lee KB, Bai LB, Yoon TR, et al. Second-look arthroscopic findings and clinical outcomes after microfracture for osteochondral lesions of the talus. Am J Sports Med 2009;37(S1):63S–70S.

23. Gomoll AH, Madry H, Knutsen G, et al. The subchondral bone in articular cartilage repair: current problems in the surgical management. Knee Surg Sports Traumatol Arthrosc 2010;18:434–47.

Arthroscopic Treatment of Anterior Ankle Impingement

Keith Jacobson, DPM[a],*, Alan Ng, DPM[a,b], Kyle E. Haffner, DPM[c]

KEYWORDS

- Ankle arthroscopy • Anterolateral ankle impingement
- Anterior ankle impingement • Chronic ankle pain
- Soft-tissue ankle impingement

Ankle impingement was first described in 1942 by Morris as athlete's ankle and was later coined footballer's ankle by McMurray.[1,2] Today, anterior ankle impingement syndrome describes the condition in which anatomic structures become entrapped in and around the ankle joint leading to chronic pain and potentially decreased range of motion. Ankle impingement can be caused by either soft-tissue or osseous pathology and is often classified by the location within the ankle joint. The most common areas of ankle impingement include anterolateral, anterior, and posterior. This article discusses common etiologies, clinical and diagnostic evaluation, treatment options, and outcomes for anterior ankle impingement.

ANTEROLATERAL ANKLE IMPINGEMENT

There are more than 23,000 inversion ankle sprains daily in the United States and it is the most frequently observed injury in athletics.[3] Approximately 20% of patients will have residual or chronic ankle pain.[3] Studies have shown that 50% of all basketball players with ankle sprains had residual symptoms, with 15% experiencing compromised playing performance.[4–6] It is estimated that 3% of all ankle sprains lead to anterolateral impingement.[7] Some think the term chronic ankle sprain should be replaced by anterolateral impingement of the ankle.[8] The 3 most common types of soft-tissue lesions that have been documented to cause anterolateral impingement are meniscoid lesions, synovitis, and distal anterior inferior tibiofibular ligament impingement.

The authors have nothing to disclose.

[a] Private Practice, Advanced Orthopedic and Sports Medicine Specialist, 8101 East Lowry Boulevard, Suite 230, Denver, CO 80230, USA
[b] Highlands Presbyterian St Luke's Podiatric Medicine and Surgery Residency Program, 1719 East 19th Avenue, 5-C East, Denver, CO 80218, USA
[c] West Houston Medical Center Podiatric Medicine and Surgery Residency Program, 12121 Richmond Avenue, Suite 417, Houston, TX 77082, USA
* Corresponding author.
E-mail address: kjacobsontx@comcast.net

Clin Podiatr Med Surg 28 (2011) 491–510
doi:10.1016/j.cpm.2011.05.002
0891-8422/11/$ – see front matter © 2011 Elsevier Inc. All rights reserved.

Meniscoid Lesion

In 1950, Wolin and colleagues[9] were the first to describe a cause for anterolateral impingement. The study consisted of 9 patients with chronic pain and swelling to the anterolateral aspect of the ankle after an inversion ankle sprain. Upon surgical examination, patients were found to have a soft-tissue mass consisting of hyalinized tissue that the investigators identified as meniscoid lesions because of its resemblance to a torn knee meniscus. These fibrous adhesions are well-developed bands of scar tissue that occur from the anterior talofibular ligament and extend into the ankle joint, resting in the lateral gutter (**Fig. 1**). Upon removal of the meniscoid lesions, Wolin noted improvement of the patient's symptoms. Initially thought to be torn ends of a ligament, histopathologic analysis revealed no ligamentous tissue.[8] Several investigators have noted and attributed meniscoid lesions to the cause of anterolateral ankle pain.[10,11]

Synovitis

Synovitis may also occur after an inversion ankle sprain.[8] The sprain may damage the anterior talofibular ligament (ATFL), anterior inferior tibiofibular ligament (AITFL), or the calcaneal fibular ligament without causing frank instability. Improper treatment and rehabilitation will lead to inadequate healing, allowing repetitive motion to cause inflammation at the ligament ends. Over time, continued activity allows the synovium to enlarge, causing impingement in the lateral gutter and chronic lateral ankle pain (**Fig. 2**).[8] Hemorrhagic synovitis can occur because of mild capsule tearing resulting in hematoma formation. The hematoma eventually is resorbed by the synovium, causing synovitis. In Ferkel and Fisher's[12] study of 31 patients with anterolateral ankle impingement, all had either hypertrophic or hemorrhagic synovitis. Subsequent studies have noted a majority of patients having synovitis present with anterolateral ankle impingement. Recently, an intraoperative classification was developed to describe impingement in the lateral gutter. This classification was based on the degree of obstruction in the lateral gutter. It ranged from normal (no abnormal soft tissue present) to severe (excessive anterolateral soft tissue preventing any visualization before shaving/debridement). In a study consisting of 41 patients with anterolateral impingement, 7 patients were noted to have what the investigators termed "synovial shelves," which was described as a hypertrophic band of synovium extending from the anterolateral aspect of the fibula over the lateral shoulder of the talus to the anterior ankle.[13] It has been noted that early resection of impinging synovium inhibits the progression of the cascade to chronic synovitis and scar-tissue formation.[14]

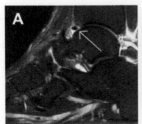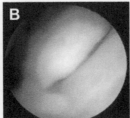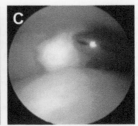

Fig. 1. Meniscoid lesion. (*A*) Sagittal T2 MRI demonstrating anterior joint effusion with a loose body (*arrow*) noted on the anterior lip of the tibia. Joint effusion with increased signal intensity is noted around os trigonum. (*B*) Arthroscopic image reveals meniscoid lesion. (*C*) After partial resection with probe demonstrating no associated articular damage.

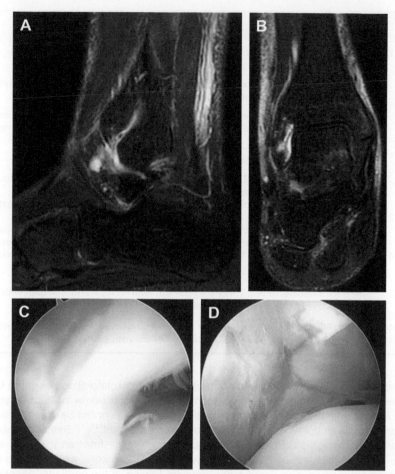

Fig. 2. MRI and arthroscopic view of anterolateral soft-tissue impingement. (*A*) Sagittal T2 demonstrating an area of intermediate signal intensity anterior to the fibula, displacing normal fat. (*B*) Coronal T2 demonstrates joint effusion in the lateral gutter of the talus. (*C*) Arthroscopic examination reveals hypertrophic synovitis causing anterolateral impingement. (*D*) After debridement of soft-tissue impingement.

Distal Fascicle of Anterior Inferior Tibiofibular Ligament (Bassett's Ligament)

Bassett and colleagues[15] discovered another cause of impingement after inversion ankle sprains when they described the distal fascicle of the AITFL. Nikoloponlous[16] originally described Bassett's ligament in 1982 as an accessory AITFL because of the distinct fibrofatty septum between the two ligaments. The research, however, was never published in the English literature.[16] The incidence of the distal fascicle of the AITFL ranges from 21% to 92%, with variation most likely caused by varying descriptions of the distal fascicle.[15–19] One investigator noted that it is most likely a common finding and only becomes pathologic after ankle mechanics become changed. The distal fascicle is found inferior and parallel to the AITFL, with its length ranging from 17 to 22 mm, a thickness of 1 to 2 mm, and width of 3 to 5 mm. An anatomic report by Ray and Kriz[19] devised a classification system describing 5 distinct types (**Box 1, Fig. 3**).

Box 1
AITFL classification system

Type 1   There are multiple fascicles (more than 3) with or without small gaps between adjacent fascicles.

A1: the inferior fascicle is separated from the rest of the ligament by a gap and possesses its own distinct proximal and distal attachments.

B1: the inferior fascicle is not completely separated from the rest of the ligament by a gap. Either its proximal or its distal attachment is continuous with the rest of the ligament.

C1: there are multiple fascicles without gaps intervening between them.

Type 2   There are 3 fascicles or less. There is a distinct inferior fascicle with both its proximal and distal attachments separate from the rest of the ligament. The inferior fascicle is separated completely from the main portion of the ligament by a gap.

Type 3   There are 3 fascicles or less. There is a distinct inferior fascicle with either its proximal or its distal attachment continuous with the rest of the ligament. A gap does not completely separate the inferior fascicle from the rest of the ligament.

Type 4   There are 3 fascicles or less. The lower portion of the ligament possesses an inferior fascicle with both its proximal and distal attachments for the rest of the ligament.

Type 5   There are 3 fascicles or less. There is a ligament with no separations or gaps within its structure. It may or may not possess a fascicular arrangement.

Adapted from Ray RG, Kriz BM. Anterior inferior tibiofibular ligament. Variations and relationship to the talus. J Am Podiatr Med Assoc 1991;81(9):479–85; with permission.

The distal fascicle runs in intimate contact with the anterolateral corner of the talus. Ray and Kriz noted lateral border impingement of the talar dome in 35 of 46 specimens. In anatomic studies, associated cartilage damage is noted between 17% and 89% and has been confirmed during arthroscopic treatment.[15–19] Bassett attributed the cartilage damage as a result of increased ankle laxity from an inversion ankle sprain.[15] The attenuation of the ATFL allows the anterior lateral aspect of the talus to extrude anteriorly during dorsiflexion, causing fraying of the cartilage. Akseki and colleagues[18] transected the ATFL in cadavers and placed the ankle through range-of-motion testing. This process led to 4 differences where distal fascicles were already in contact with the talus in a neutral position (42 of 47 specimens).

The variation of width, length, and obliquity may also be related to pathology. Akseki determined that the mean width and length were significantly higher in fascicles that bent during dorsiflexion. It was also noted that the more distal the insertion of the fascicle near the ATFL, the more often impingement occurred.[19] Bassett noted that bending of the fascicle on dorsiflexion greater than 12° might be the source of thickening and impingement. It has been noted that manual distraction of the ankle joint relieves contact and impingement of the fascicle on the talus.[15] Therefore, the investigators concluded that the use of intraoperative distraction might cause the surgeon to miss a pathologic distal fascicle (**Fig. 4**).

ANTERIOR ANKLE IMPINGEMENT

Anterior ankle impingement is most commonly caused by an osseous etiology presenting as pain in the anterior medial aspect of the ankle. Although there are small case studies of soft tissue and space occupying lesions causing anterior ankle impingement (**Fig. 5**), this section focuses on osseous pathology.[20,21]

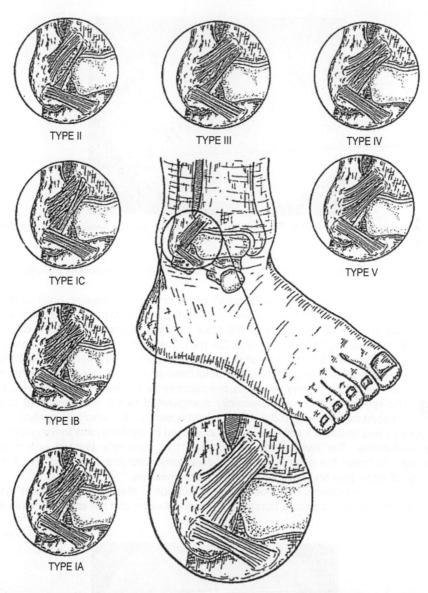

Fig. 3. Anatomic classification system of distal anterior inferior tibiofibular ligament devised by Ray and Kriz. (*From* Ray RG, Kriz BM. Anterior inferior tibiofibular ligament. Variations and relationship to the talus. J Am Podiatr Med Assoc 1991;81:482; with permission.)

Osseous

Formation of tibiotalar osteophytes at the anterior aspect of the ankle is a common cause of chronic ankle pain.[22] Anterior ankle spurring is a common occurrence in the athletic community, ranging from 45% to 60%.[23] Historically, 2 hypotheses for the etiology of anterior osteophyte formation have been described. According to McMurray,[2] anterior osteophyte formation develops from repeated capsular traction while having the foot in a maximally plantar-flexed position. The investigator used the example of an athlete kicking a soccer ball. Other investigators have supported

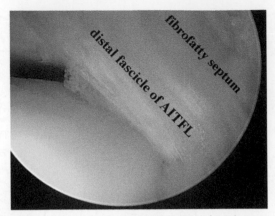

Fig. 4. Arthroscopic view of AITFL with associated distal fascicle separated by fibrofatty septum.

this theory. However, recent anatomic studies have demonstrated this hypothesis to be unfeasible.[24]

One cadaveric study measured the width of the non–weight-bearing tibial cartilage rim, and the distance from the tibial and talar cartilage from capsular structures were measured. The results revealed that the tibial cartilage to capsule distance was 4.3 mm and talar cartilage to capsule was 2.4 mm. The width of the tibial non–weight-bearing cartilage was 2.4 mm. This study refutes the theory that osteophyte formation is caused by traction.[24] Arthroscopically, tibial osteophytes are noted to be within the joint, and it is not necessary to reflect the capsule to remove the osteophyte. The cadaveric specimens were also manually manipulated to 15° dorsiflexion to study the soft-tissue components at the anterior joint space. Histopathologic analysis was performed and revealed a soft-tissue layer bordered by synovial cells forming a synovial membrane. The investigators concluded that anteriorly located soft tissue impinges between the osteophytes. This soft tissue becomes inflamed and is the source of ankle pain and not the osteophytes themselves.

The second hypothesis described by O'Donoghue,[25] states that the osteophytes were caused by direct trauma during forcible dorsiflexion and not at extreme plantar

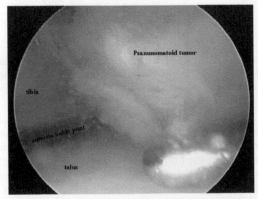

Fig. 5. Arthroscopic view of anterolateral ankle impingement caused from psammomatoid tumor.

flexion causing traction as initially stated by McMurray. The author noted patients to have pain on end range of dorsiflexion or as the author coined "drive."[25] Stoller and colleagues[23] theorized that repeated impingement causes subperiosteal hemorrhages and subsequent bone growth.

It has been noted that the non–weight-bearing anterior cartilage rim undergoes osteophytic transformation.[26] The investigator thought the osteophyte formation was caused by direct damage and recurrent microtrauma to the anterior cartilage rim. The same investigators performed a biomechanical analysis to determine if whether kicking a soccer ball could cause osteophyte formation by hyperplantar flexion or by direct impact.[22] Results revealed that in 39% of kicking movements, maximum plantar flexion exceeded the subject's static maximum plantar flexion. The soccer ball impact was noted at the anterior part of the medial malleolus in 76% of ball strikes, with ball velocity averaging 24.6 m/s and contact force of 1025 N. The investigators concluded that the impact location and force, not extreme plantar flexion, support the hypothesis that spur formation occurs from direct repetitive trauma to the anterior cartilage rim. This microtrauma may be compounded in patients with a history of supination injuries. A history of supination injuries has also been documented in 76% of patients with osteophyte formation in one study, and in another study the incidence of spurs was 3 times higher in an unstable ankle joint compared with a group without ankle instability.[27]

CLINICAL PRESENTATION

Patients typically present complaining of a prolonged and persistent pain in the ankle with a history of a recent traumatic event. Patients are usually younger athletes who have a history of an inversion ankle sprain in which symptoms have not resolved. Patients may state that they have had multiple ankle sprains or may describe just 1 serious traumatic occurrence.

Typically, patients have increased pain after prolonged walking or physical activity. Patients may also describe a popping or catching within the ankle joint.

Physical examination reveals pain on palpation along the anterior lateral aspect of the talus, the lateral gutter, and the most inferior aspect of the tibiofibular articulation. Soft-tissue swelling is present in the anterolateral shoulder of the ankle joint and palpable masses are occasionally noted within the lateral gutter.[9] Pain can be elicited with passive dorsiflexion and eversion. An audible click may also be heard during ankle range of motion. This click has been attributed to AITFL impingement. The "ankle impingement sign," described by Malloy, uses thumb pressure over the lateral gutter while taking the ankle from a plantar-flexed position to maximal dorsiflexion. The investigators noted that if hypertrophic synovitis is present, this maneuver impinges the synovium between the neck of the talus and the distal tibia. This test has been reported to be 94.8% sensitive and 88.0% specific for synovial hypertrophy.[28]

Liu and colleagues[29] noted 94% sensitivity and 75% specificity predicting anterolateral ankle impingement using their clinical examination. Impingement was considered positive when at least 5 of 6 clinical parameters were present:

- Anterolateral ankle joint tenderness
- Anterolateral joint swelling
- Pain with forced dorsiflexion and eversion
- Pain with single-leg squat
- Pain with activities
- Absence of instability.

The clinician must rule out other causes of anterior lateral ankle pain, such as osteo-chondral lesions of the talus, peroneal tendonitis or subluxation, tarsal coalitions, and subtalar joint dysfunction.[30]

In anterior ankle impingement, patients will describe pain on dorsiflexion with a subjective feeling of stopping or blocked dorsiflexion. McMurray[2] observed patients having pain and difficulty kicking a soccer ball correctly at the medial aspect of the ankle. Pain was not elicited when the ball was kicked improperly with the toes. Ballet dancers will describe pain in demi-plié or grand-plié and with landing from a leap.[31] On physical examination, pain on palpation is noted to the medial aspect of the ankle joint. With the foot in maximum plantar flexion, osteophytes may be palpable medial to the tibialis anterior tendon or along the anterior rim of the tibia because of the thin subcu-taneous tissue.[26]

Radiographic Evaluation

In patients with anterolateral impingement, plain radiographs should be performed to rule out fractures, widening of the ankle mortise, or arthritic changes. Stress radio-graphs can be used to rule out ligament laxity. In patients with suspected anterior ankle impingement, accurate detection and localization of spurs are necessary for preoperative planning.[26] Standard anteroposterior and lateral views should be per-formed to detect anterior tibial and talar spurring. Scranton and McDermott[32] devised a classification for spur formation: stage I, osteophyte less than 3 mm; stage II, osteo-phyte greater than 3 mm; stage III, anterior tibial osteophyte with talar osteophyte (kissing lesion); and stage IV, panarthritis. Standard lateral films have been shown to be capable of detecting only 40% of tibial and 32% of talar osteophytes. The ante-romedial notch and anteromedial contour can inhibit the detection of anteromedial osteophytes.[33] Tol and colleagues[33] devised an oblique radiograph (45/30 anterome-dial impingement [AMI] view) where the beam is tilted 45° in the craniocaudal direction with the leg in 30° of external rotation and the foot plantar flexed. In a study of 60 patients with anterior impingement, lateral radiographs were only able to detect lateral spurring in 58% of ankles. When detecting both tibial and talar osteophytes, the lateral view was 40% and 32% sensitive. When combined with the 45/30 AMI view, sensitivity increased to 85% and 73%.

Magnetic Resonance Imaging

Radiographic evaluation is essential for determining osseous pathology. Magnetic reso-nance imaging (MRI) is the most useful imaging modality for evaluating soft-tissue impingement or excluding other ankle pathologies, such as osteochondral defects, pero-neal tendonitis, tarsal coalitions, and sinus tarsi syndrome.[34] The literature for MRI effi-cacy for diagnosis of anterolateral soft-tissue impingement varies immensely with sensitivities ranging from 39% to 100% and specificities from 50% to 100%.[12,29,34–42]

In 1991, Ferkel's[8] study had 3 patients that showed increased signal intensity in the lateral gutter with the use of MRI. The investigator noted MRI might be beneficial. In early studies, many investigators failed to use MRI because of the lack of sensitivity and accuracy and because they thought it was an unnecessary expense.[9,43] Liu and colleagues[29] compared clinical examination versus MRI evaluation of 22 patients with chronic anterolateral ankle pain. The results revealed 94% sensitivity and 75% specificity for clinical examination compared with MRI, which had 39% sensitivity and 50% specificity.

Rubin's[39] review of 18 patients with arthroscopically confirmed ankle impingement revealed 9 of the 18 patients had ankle effusion in the lateral gutter. Eight of these patients had a soft-tissue mass noted in the lateral recess. In the remaining 9 patients, no joint effusion was noted and soft-tissue masses were not appreciated. The investigator concluded that without joint effusion a diagnosis of impingement could not be determined.

In a study of 12 patients with anterolateral impingement, MR images were reviewed for presence of lateral gutter fullness and ATFL thickening. An additional 20 ankles (19 subjects) without an impingement diagnosis were used as a control.[41] The rate of thickening of the ATFL and lateral gutter fullness were noted to be higher in patients with impingement, however, it was not statistically significant. Sensitivity, specificity, and accuracy for the diagnosis of impingement was noted to be 42%, 85%, and 69%, respectively, with the investigator concluding that lateral gutter fullness and ATFL thickening may be suggestive of impingement, but the reliability is questionable.

Duncan retrospectively reviewed 24 patients with preoperative MRI who underwent ankle arthroscopy.[37] Twelve patients were known to have anterolateral impingement with a control group comprised of 12 subjects. The results by 3 reviewers revealed sensitivities of 75% to 83% and specificities of 75% to 100%. The investigator concluded MRI should not be used as the sole diagnostic tool and will not replace a thorough history and physical examination but serves as a valuable adjunct to access overall ankle pathology. In Ferkel's[12] most recent study, MRI evaluation of anterolateral impingement revealed a sensitivity and specificity of 83.3% and 78.6%, respectively, with an accuracy of 79%. Of the 24 patients, 14 (58%) had other associated diagnoses that were found during MRI evaluation that did not involve the lateral impingement, allowing an alteration in the surgical plan for 8 patients. The investigator advocated the use of MRI in patients with a complicated presentation, which may allow exclusion or inclusion of other pathology.

MRI Characteristics

Axial T-1 weighted or proton-density weighted images combined with sagittal T-1 weighted images have been shown to be the most accurate for identification of pathology. Findings on axial images may reveal fullness in the anterolateral gutter and a focal mass within the gutter. The mass has low signal intensity on T1 images and low to moderate signal intensity on T2 images.[12] Evaluation of the ATFL can also be observed on axial images with thickening or nodularity being present. Syndesmotic pathology will appear as a thickened soft-tissue mass with low signal intensity on T1 axial images (**Fig. 6**).[34,35,38] Synovitis is manifested as either linear or a conglomerate foci with intermediate signal intensity on T-2 weighted and fat-suppressed proton density axial images. The use of sagittal T1-images and short-tau inversion recovery images have recently been shown to be effective in diagnosis of anterolateral ankle impingement.[12,37] On sagittal T1-weighted images, superficial fat is normally directly adjacent to the fibula. The joint capsule appears contiguous and the ATFL is noted to be thin and homogenous in signal intensity. Pathology is noted when an abnormal area of low signal intensity is displacing the normal fat from the anterior aspect of the fibula (see **Fig. 2**).[12]

In most cases, radiographic evaluation is adequate to detect and locate tibiotalar exostoses. MRI is not indicated unless other associated soft-tissue pathology is suspected. When used, MRI can accurately locate spurs as well as adjacent synovitis, fibrosis, and capsular thickening on sagittal T1-weighted imaging (**Fig. 7**).[34,35] Sagittal T2-weighted imaging reveals subchondral bone marrow edema and joint effusion. When the tibial plafond exostosis demonstrates enlargement inferiorly, it may impinge on the talar dome articular cartilage. This impingement causes a tram-track–type chondral lesion on the talar dome.[34,35] These lesions are best seen on sagittal T1-weighted or proton-density weighted images.[35]

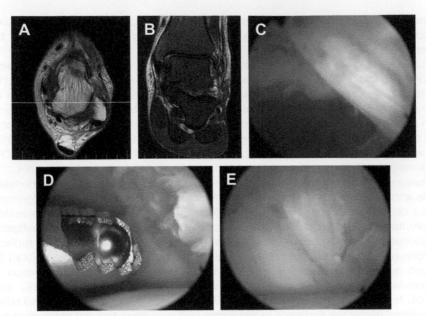

Fig. 6. MRI and arthroscopic examination demonstrating hypertrophic distal AITFL. (*A*) Axial cut T1 and (*B*) sagittal T2 images reveal a hypertrophic AITFL. Arthroscopic examination reveals before (*C*), during (*D*), and after (*E*) debridement.

Magnetic Resonance Arthrography

Direct MR arthrography (MRA) with the injection of diluted gadolinium solution may be beneficial in the identification of ligament tears in the ankle and it also increases the sensitivity for diagnosis of ankle impingement syndrome.[44] MRA has been found to be accurate (97%), sensitive (96%), and specific (100%) for the diagnosis of anterolateral impingement. Findings include focal or irregular soft-tissue nodularity and thickening between the AITFL and the ATFL. A lack of normal joint distention in the anterolateral gutter is most likely caused by scar-tissue formation and adhesions at the fibula, preventing fluid from entering the normal recess. According to Robinson,[40] this finding was always associated with scarring and synovitis upon arthroscopic examination.[40] MRA, however, is a minimally invasive procedure that requires needle

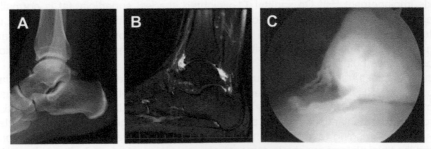

Fig. 7. Radiographic (*A*), MRI (*B*), and arthroscopic view (*C*) of bony anterior ankle impingement. Lateral radiograph (*A*) reveals an osteophyte on both tibia and talus. Sagittal T2 imaging (*B*) allows visualization of ankle effusion as well as offending osteophyte. Arthroscopic view (*C*) of anterior tibial osteophyte predebridement.

placement into the joint under fluoroscopy and noted to be expensive.[35] Others have discussed the use of indirect MRA in which gadodiamide is injected intravenously to observe impingement pathology.[44] The synovial membrane is normally highly vascular. Inflammation of the synovium has increased vascularity, allowing for greater uptake, therefore, contrast is noted to be superior to conventional MRI in delineating structures where minimal joint effusion is noted.[44] However, studies have shown little to no additional value in detection of ankle impingement compared with conventional MRI.

Computed Tomography

Computed tomography (CT) is useful in the analysis of osseous and cartilaginous pathology, such as loose bodies, chondral and osteochondral lesions of the talar dome, and degenerative joint disease. The use of CT arthrography has been shown to be useful for the diagnosis of soft-tissue impingement. Hauger and colleagues[45] evaluated 44 patients with chronic ankle pain who underwent arthroscopic treatment. CT arthrography revealed 4 types of patterns in the anterolateral compartment of the ankle. Type 0 and I patterns were noted to be consistent with normal anatomy. Type II and III patterns consisted of abnormal pathology. Type II lesions were identified as nodular thickening of the capsule producing a double rim at the level of the lateral groove. On arthroscopic analysis of the 11 type II lesions, 10 were noted to be meniscoid bodies (91% sensitivity). Type III lesions appeared as an abundant fibrous reaction with frayed appearance at the level of the lateral groove. Arthroscopically, 100% of 14 patients were noted to have an inflammatory process. It was also noted that 16 of 26 patients with impingement had an associated osteochondral lesion. The investigators noted that CT arthrography could be considered the gold standard in the analysis of chronic ankle pain given the high sensitivity for the diagnosis of bone, cartilage, and soft-tissue lesions.[45]

The use of 3-dimensional (3D) CT has been shown to be of use in the preoperative planning for arthroscopic removal of anterior tibiotalar osteophytes.[46] Takao and colleagues[46] evaluated 16 patients with tibiotalar osteophytes with 3D CT to investigate the size, shape, location, and number of osteophytes for preoperative planning. There were 5 subjects used as a control in which 3D CT was not used in preoperative planning. Postoperative scores were 96.8 in the 3D CT group and 88.5 in the control group. The investigators concluded that 3D CT is useful to thoroughly remove all osteophytes and obtain excellent clinical results in later-stage osteophyte formation.

TREATMENT
Conservative

Initial management of anterior impingement involves conservative measures, such as oral antiinflammatory medications, ice, corticosteroid injections, orthoses, heel lifts, and physical therapy. Physical therapy modalities consist of ultrasound, electrical stimulation, range-of-motion exercises, proprioceptive training, and strengthening exercises. Patients who fail to respond to conservative treatment and continue to experience pain and decrease range of motion after 3 to 6 months are potential surgical candidates.[47]

TECHNIQUE

The following is a brief discussion of the technique employed by authors KJ and AN when approaching all types of anterior ankle impingement. Initially, patients are placed in the supine position with the knees directly adjacent to the bend in the foot of the table. A thigh tourniquet is used. Before prepping the surgical site, the ankle joint is insufflated with approximately 10 to 15 mL of 0.5% bupivacaine hydrochloride (Marcaine) with epinephrine.

Some surgeons use distraction, however, the authors find that distraction is not necessary when addressing this pathology alone. If one choses, invasive and noninvasive distraction is available.

Two portals are typically sufficient to address all types of anterior ankle impingement. The anteromedial and anterolateral portals are routinely used. The anteromedial portal is first created by placing a small stab incision directly medial to the tibialis anterior tendon adjacent to the ankle joint. The stab incision is made in the dermis only, and further dissection to the joint capsule is performed using a mosquito. With the mosquito separating the tissue, a blunt trocar and cannula are inserted through the capsule and into the ankle joint. Inflow is provided through this cannula using gravity or a pressure pump. The camera is then inserted, allowing direct visualization of the joint. The authors use a 4.0-mm scope, but a 2.7-mm scope is available. The anterolateral portal is placed just lateral to the peroneus tertius tendon. Special care must be taken to avoid the neurovascular structures. This approach can be aided by illuminating the anterolateral portal area with the inserted camera. The same technique to create the anteromedial portal is repeated for the anterolateral portal. However, only a blunt trocar is inserted to create the portal. The cannula is removed to allow placement of whatever ancillary equipment (incisors, bone cutters, burrs, electrocautery, and so forth) will be used to remove the offending pathology. The outflow is provided through the ancillary instrumentation. If one finds difficulty removing the pathology given the previous setup, the camera can be switched to the anterolateral portal with the resection instrumentation placed through the anteromedial portal.

After the pathology is removed, the ankle joint is irrigated and all instrumentation is removed. A 5-0 nylon is used to close the dermis only, and the portal sites and ankle joint are anesthetized locally. A dry sterile dressing is applied and a protective boot is placed. Depending on the pathology, patients are typically full weight bearing but may be placed non–weight bearing for 1 to 2 weeks. Range of motion of the ankle joint should begin as soon as is feasible.

CLINICAL STUDIES

Reports detailing arthroscopic treatment of ankle impingement from soft-tissue pathology that failed conservative treatment have consistently favorable results, with excellent to good results ranging from 75% to 96% (**Table 1**).[8,10,11,13,14,48–54] Martin had the first study with extended follow-up of patients with soft-tissue anterior ankle impingement. The investigators reported good to excellent outcomes in 12 of 16 patients after a 2-year follow-up.[10] Ferkel and colleagues[8] retrospectively reviewed 31 patients with greater than a 2-year follow-up. The results revealed 85% good to excellent outcomes. Continuing with successful outcomes, a review by Meislin and colleagues[14] of 29 patients with synovial impingement yielded 90% good to excellent outcome at the 25-month follow-up using the same scoring system as Ferkel and Martin.

DeBerardino[48] retrospectively studied a homogenous group of military men and women with an average age of 24 years. All 60 patients with anterolateral ankle impingement were involved in competitive athletics. The results of this study using the West Point Ankle score system revealed 96% good to excellent outcomes.[48]

In more recent studies using the American Orthopaedic Foot and Ankle Society (AOFAS) ankle score system, Urguden and colleagues[13] reported outcomes on 41 patients with a mean follow-up of 84 months.[13] The investigators used both the Meislin and AOFAS ankle scores for 37 good to excellent and an average AOFAS score of

Table 1
Arthroscopic treatment of anterior ankle impingement (soft tissue)

Author/Year	Evidence	Sample Size	Follow-Up (mo)	Outcome	Comment
Martin et al,[10] 1989	IV	16	25–40	12 good to excellent (75%)	—
Ferkel et al,[8] 1991	IV	31	33.5	Good to excellent (85%)	Weber ankle scoring scale
Meislin et al,[14] 1993	IV	29	25	26 good to excellent (90%)	Weber ankle scoring scale (modified)
DeBerardino et al,[48] 1997	IV	60	27	58 good to excellent (96%)	West Point Ankle scoring
Kim and Ha,[52] 2000	II	52	30	49 good to excellent (94%)	2 groups: group I (stable ankle), group II (unstable ankle); no statistical significance between groups
Rasmussen and Hjorth Jensen,[50] 2002	IV	105	24	92 good to excellent (88%)	Both bony and soft-tissue impingement
Gulish et al,[49] 2005	IV	11	25	10/11 good to excellent (91%)	Adolescents aged 13–19 y AOFAS 95
Urguden et al,[13] 2005	IV	41	84	36 good to excellent (88%)	AOFAS 89.6; chondral lesions resulted in poorer outcome
Baums et al,[59] 2006	III	12	31	Karlsson score 90	28-point increase from preoperative Karlsson score; no statistical difference from osteophyte group
Hassan[51] 2007	IV	23	25	21 good to excellent (91%)	AOFAS 89
El-Sayed[53] 2010	IV	20	21	17 good to excellent (85%)	5 patients with AITFL injuries; poorer outcome in patients with syndesmotic and chondral lesions

89.6. In Hasaan's prospective study of 23 patients with anterolateral ankle impingement, the preoperative AOFAS ankle score was 34 (range 4–57), with a postoperative AOFAS score, after an average follow-up of 25 months, of 89 (range 60–100).[51] El-Sayed[53] reported good to excellent results in 17 of 20 (85%) patients, with an average Japanese Society of Surgery of the Foot score increase by 39 points (preoperative 46.8, postoperative 86.5).

There has been much discussion and debate concerning outcomes in patients with soft-tissue ankle impingement associated with intraarticular pathology and ankle instability. Multiple studies have shown that chondral lesions and ankle instability do not affect patient outcomes.[15,48] Both Deberardino[48] and Bassett[15] found that chondral lesions did not affect outcomes. In Deberardino's study, 17 patients had both soft-tissue ankle impingement with chondromalacia of either the talus or tibia. These 17 patients all had good to excellent outcomes. When compared with patients without chondral lesions, no statistical significance was noted. El-Sayed had 7 (35%) patients with associated cartilage pathology, the investigator stated that there was no statistical significance between patients with cartilage damage and those without.[53] The conclusion by the investigator concerning the reason that there was no statistical significance between groups was because of the apparent superficial nature of cartilage damage (grade I and II).

In contrast to these studies, others have noted intraarticular pathology as a cause for poorer outcomes. Ferkel's initial study had 4 patients with fair results. Three of these patients had grade II chondromalacia of the talus and reported constant ankle pain.[8] One study[51] had 4 patients with cartilage damage, and AOFAS scores were significantly lower (83) compared with the group without intraarticular pathology (91). Urguden had 19 patients with anterolateral talar dome grade III chondromalacia. AOFAS ankle scores were significantly different between ankles with concomitant intraarticular pathology and those without; 83.0 compared with 96.65 respectively. Of the 19 patients, there were 2 excellent and 13 good results. However, in the remaining 21 patients without instability or chondral lesion resulted in 18 excellent and 3 good results.[13]

The correlation between repeated inversion ankle injuries and instability of the syndesmosis has been documented.[13,52] Meislin and colleagues[14] had 3 patients with ankle instability in which all were graded with fair results.[14] They noted that after lateral ankle reconstruction, patients were free of instability and pain. The investigators concluded that patients with ankle instability should have ankle reconstruction as their initial treatment. Urguden noted syndesmotic instability arthroscopically in 3 patients. Two of these patients resulted in poor results, with AOFAS scores of 60 and 65, respectively.[13] A recent study[53] had 3 patients with an AITFL tear, and postoperatively recurrent inversion ankle sprains occurred. These previous studies are small in nature compared with Kim and Ha's[52] prospective review of anterolateral soft-tissue impingement. A total of 52 patients were stressed with a Telos device (METAX, Germany) and then divided equally into 2 groups with and without ankle instability. No attempt was made to primarily repair the group with instability. Results after the 30-month follow-up revealed 49 patients with good to excellent results and 3 patients with fair results. Comparing the 2 groups revealed no statistical significance.

In the adolescent population, anterolateral impingement may occur after ankle sprains. One study demonstrated that ankle sprains are more prevalent from the ages of 15 to 19 years.[54] Gulish and colleagues[49] reviewed 12 patients, aged between 13 and 19 years, arthroscopically treated for chronic anterolateral ankle pain. All patients were diagnosed with functional instability with a Telos stress device. The postoperative average AOFAS score was 95, with results ranging from 75 to 100.[49] Edmonds and colleagues[54] studied 13 adolescent patients by evaluating the nonoperative management of anterolateral ankle impingement versus immediate surgical management. Patients were all given an initial course of physical therapy of at least 6 weeks; at this time, none of the patients were able to return to sports because of continued pain, and they went on to surgical intervention. AOFAS scores were obtained at the initial visit after physical therapy and at the final surgical follow-up. The patients' initial AOFAS rating was 68.4. After a mean of 6 months of nonoperative treatment and physical therapy, the AOFAS rating was 68.2. At the final follow-up visit, after ankle arthroscopy for anterolateral impingement, the final AOFAS score 90.6. The investigators concluded that after clinical diagnosis of impingement is confirmed, no significant improvement occurs with nonsurgical treatment. In both studies combined, of the 25 adolescent patients treated, 22 were girls. Gulish noted adolescent girls may be more prone to ankle impingement than boys, which would be in line with other sports-related injuries, such as anterior cruciate ligament tears.

Two studies have compared soft-tissue and bony impingement for anterior ankle impingement (see **Table 1; Table 2**).[11,50] In a prospective review, Baums and colleagues[11] studied 26 athletes with soft-tissue (12 patients) and bony impingement (14 patients). Patients were evaluated on the Karlsson ankle score, visual analog scale, and Tenger activity score. There was no statistical significance in outcome between the two groups. Both groups' Karlsson ankle score improved significantly by 28 and 33 points, respectively (see **Figs. 1** and **2**). At 24-months follow-up, 25 of the patients returned to full activities in their respective sports.[11] In a prospective study by Rasmussen and Jensen,[50] 105 patients were treated arthroscopically for anterior ankle pain.[50] In 177 diagnoses, a diagnosis of soft-tissue impingement was made 89 times, and 44 times in anterior bony impingement. At a follow-up of 24 months, 92 patients had good to excellent results, with improvement of ankle range of motion and reduction in pain noted.

One of the earliest studies on bony anterior ankle impingement was performed by Scranton and McDermott[32] in which the investigators compared treatment outcomes of open ankle arthrotomy versus ankle arthroscopy (see **Table 2**). This study was comprised of 37 patients (43 ankles). The investigators, however, did not randomize the treatment groups. The treatment groups were compared on operating room time, recovery time, and length of hospitalization. Results revealed operating room time was the same between the two groups; however, recovery time was half the length, and return to athletics was 1 month faster in the arthroscopy-treated group. There was a direct correlation between severity of the bony impingement and recovery rate. Grade II spurs recovered on average in 5.6 weeks as compared to 10 weeks for grade IV spurs. Ogilvie-Harris studied 17 patients with painful limited ankle range of motion caused by anterior bone impingement.[55] Patients' symptoms were graded on range of motion of the ankle joint and five specific parameters both preoperatively and postoperatively. At the 39-month follow-up, 92% of patients had good to excellent outcomes, and ankle dorsiflexion increased from 3° to 12°. In a study of 13 athletes with bony impingement, 10 patients were able to return to preoperative sports at 14 weeks, and there was a 92% good to excellent outcome for the study (see **Table 2**).[56]

Van Dijk and colleagues[26,57] determined that there was a difference between patients' results when joint space narrowing is involved. In an initial study presented by Van Dijk and colleagues,[26] 62 patients with bony anterior ankle impingement were preoperatively classified into 4 grades utilizing radiographic findings (**Table 3**). At the 2-year postoperative follow-up, all patients' pain and function were significantly better, with an initial visual analog scale (VAS) score of 6.3 compared with the final follow-up score of 4.3. In patients who had osteophytes without joint space narrowing

Table 2
Arthroscopic treatment of anterior ankle impingement (bone)

Author/Year	Evidence	Sample Size	Follow-Up	Outcome	Comment
Scranton & McDermott,[32] 1992	IV	43 ankle	36 mo	Relief of symptoms and pain	Arthroscopy group versus arthrotomy group; arthroscopy group recovered in 5 weeks compared to 8 weeks
Ogilvie-Harris et al,[55] 1993	IV	17	39 mo	16 good to excellent	Points graded on 5 parameters (swelling, pain, stiffness, activity, and limping)
Reynaert et al,[56] 1994	IV	13	19 mo	Good to excellent (92%)	10 patients returned to sports at 14 weeks
Van Dijk et al,[26] 1997	IV	62	24 mo	Good to excellent (73%)	Patients without joint space narrowing had better outcomes compared to more advanced arthritic ankles
Tol et al,[57] 2001	IV	57	65 y	32 good to excellent (77%)	Good to excellent 77% patients without OA; good to excellent 53% patients with grade I–II OA
Takao et al,[46] 2004	IV	16	32 mo	16 good to excellent	AOFAS postoperative score 97.0; investigators used 3D CT for preoperative planning
Baums et al,[59] 2006	III	14	31 mo	Karlsson score 93	33-point increase from preoperative Karlsson score; no statistical difference from soft-tissue group

Abbreviation: OA, osteoarthritis.

Table 3
Classification for osteoarthritic changes of the ankle joint

Grade	Characteristics
0	Normal joint or subchondral sclerosis
I	Osteophytes without joint space narrowing
II	Joint space narrowing with or without osteophytes
III	(Sub)total disappearance/deformation of the joint space

Adapted from van Dijk CN, Tol JL, Verheyen CC. A prospective study of prognostic factors concerning the outcome of arthroscopic surgery for anterior ankle impingement. Am J Sports Med 1997;25(6):737–45; with permission.

(grade 0/I), there was a significant reduction in pain (VAS 7.0 to 2.5 at 2-year follow-up). Patient satisfaction was 82% good/excellent. The investigators determined that osteophytes without joint space narrowing are not a manifestation of osteoarthritis, and is essentially a normal joint when spurring has been removed. This patient population was then reviewed at the 5- to 8-year follow-up.[57] Results of the 57 patients showed that the 10 patients with grade 0 remained without osteoarthritis and had good or excellent results. Osteophytes returned in two-thirds of the patients from group I, but good to excellent results were noted in 77%. The investigators concluded that arthroscopic treatment of bony anterior osteophytes removes pain even with osteophytic recurrence.

Complications

Ferkel and colleagues[58] reported an overall complication rate of 10% in 518 patients with arthroscopically treated ankles. Neurologic complications were most common with involvement of the superficial peroneal nerve (56%), the sural nerve (24%), and the saphenous nerve (20%). In a review of the literature for this article, neurologic complications occurred most often. Infection was noted as another complication, with most being superficial in nature. In one study, the incidence of deep infection was 4%.[50] The investigators noted that all infections resolved after synovectomy and intravenous antibiotic treatment. The use of preoperative intravenous antibiosis was not used in this study. In another study, there was 1 patient that developed a deep infection after hemarthrosis. These investigators now use local anesthetic with epinephrine, preoperatively. Superficial wound dehiscence was also noted in small numbers.[47,48,51,53,54] For a complete review of the complications in ankle arthroscopy, please review the corresponding article by Chris Lamy in this issue.

REFERENCES

1. Morris LH. Report of cases of athlete's ankle. J Bone Joint Surg 1943;25:220.
2. McMurray TP. Footballer's ankle. J Bone Joint Surg 1950;32:68–9.
3. Balduni FC, Tetzlaff J. Historical perspectives on injuries of the ligaments of the ankle. Clin Sports Med 1982;1(1):3–12.
4. Liu S, Jason W. Lateral ankle sprains and instability problems. Clin Sports Med 1994;13(4):793–809.
5. Brand RL, Collins MD, Templeton T. Surgical repair of ruptured lateral ankle ligaments. Am J Sports Med 1981;9:40–4.
6. Garrick JG. Epidemiologic perspective. Clin Sports Med 1982;1:13–8.
7. Van Dijk CN. Ankle impingement. In: Chan KM, Karlsson J, editors. ISAKOS/FIMS World consensus conference on ankle instability. Hong Kong; 2005.
8. Ferkel RD, Karzel RP, Del Pizzo W, et al. Arthroscopic treatment of anterolateral impingement of the ankle. Am J Sports Med 1991;19(5):440–6.
9. Wolin I, Glassman F, Sideman S. Internal derangement of the talofibular component of the ankle. Surg Gynecol Obstet 1950;91:193–200.
10. Martin DF, Curl WW, Baker CL. Arthroscopic treatment of chronic synovitis of the ankle. Arthroscopy 1989;5:110–4.
11. Baums MH, Kahl E, Schultz W, et al. Clinical outcome of the arthroscopic management of sports-related "anterior ankle pain": a prospective study. Knee Surg Sports Traumatol Arthrosc 2004;14:482–6.
12. Ferkel RD, Tyorkin M, Applegate G, et al. MRI evaluation of anterolateral soft tissue impingement of the ankle. Foot Ankle Int 2004;31:655–61.

13. Urguden M, Soyuncu Y, Ozdemir H, et al. Arthroscopic treatment of anterolateral soft tissue impingement of the ankle: evaluation of factors affecting outcome. Arthroscopy 2005;21:317–22.

14. Meislin RJ, Rose DJ, Parisien JS, et al. Arthroscopic treatment of synovial impingement of the ankle. Am J Sports Med 1993;21:186–9.

15. Bassett FH, Gates HS, Billys JB, et al. Talar impingement by the anteroinferior tibiofibular ligament. A cause of chronic pain in the ankle after inversion sprain. J Bone Joint Surg Am 1990;72:55–9.

16. Nikolopoulos CE, Tsirikos AI, Sourmelis S, et al. The accessory anteroinferior tibiofibular ligament as a cause of talar impingement. A cadaveric study. Am J Sports Med 2004;32(2):389–95.

17. Van den Bekerom MP, Raven E. The distal fascicle of the anterior inferior tibiofibular ligament as a cause of tibiotalar impingement syndrome: a current concepts review. Knee Surg Sports Traumatol Arthrosc 2007;15:465–71.

18. Akseki D, Pinar H, Yaldiz K, et al. The anterior tibiofibular ligament and talar impingement: a cadaveric study. Knee Surg Sports Traumatol Arthrosc 2002; 10:321–6.

19. Ray RG, Kriz BM. Anterior inferior tibiofibular ligament. Variations and relationship to the talus. J Am Podiatr Med Assoc 1991;81:479–85.

20. Ergol K, Parisien S. Impingement syndrome of the ankle caused by a medial meniscoid lesion. Arthroscopy 1997;13(4):522–5.

21. Mosier- La Clair SM, Monroe MT, Manoli A. Medial impingement syndrome of the anterior tibiotalar fascicle of the deltoid ligament of the talus. Foot Ankle Int 2000; 21:385–91.

22. Tol JL, Slim E, van Soest AJ, et al. The relationship of the kicking action in soccer and anterior ankle impingement syndrome. A biomechanical analysis. Am J Sports Med 2002;30:45–50.

23. Stoller SM, Hekmat F, Kleiger B. A comparative study of the frequency of anterior impingement exostoses of the ankle in dancer and non-dancer. Foot Ankle 1984; 4:201.

24. Tol JL, van Dijk CN. Etiology of the anterior ankle impingement syndrome: a descriptive anatomical study. Foot Ankle Int 2004;25:382–6.

25. O'Donoghue DH. Impingement exostoses of the talus and tibia. J Bone Joint Surg Am 1957;39:835–52, 26.

26. van Dijk CN, Tol JL, Verheyen CC. A prospective study of prognostic factors concerning the outcome of arthroscopic surgery for anterior ankle impingement. Am J Sports Med 1997;25:737–45.

27. Scranton PE, McDermott J, Rogers J. The relationship between chronic ankle instability and variations in mortise anatomy and impingement spurs. Foot Ankle Int 2000;21(8):657–64.

28. Molloy S, Solan MC, Bendall SP. Synovial impingement in the ankle. J Bone Joint Surg Br 2003;85(3):330.

29. Liu SH, Nuccion SL, Finerman G. Diagnosis of anterolateral ankle impingement: comparison between magnetic resonance imaging and clinical examination. Am J Sports Med 1997;25(3):390–4.

30. DiGiovanni B, Fraga C, Cohen B, et al. Associated injuries found in chronic lateral ankle instability. Foot Ankle Int 2000;21(10):810.

31. Nihal A, Rose D, Trepman E. Arthroscopic treatment of anterior impingement syndrome in dancers. Foot Ankle Int 2005;26(11):908.

32. Scranton PE Jr, McDermott JE. Anterior tibiotalar spurs: a comparison of open versus arthroscopic debridement. Foot Ankle 1992;13(3):125–9.

33. Tol JL, Verhagen RA, Krips R, et al. The anterior ankle impingement syndrome: diagnostic value of oblique radiographs. Foot Ankle Int 2004;25(2):63–8.

34. Sanders T, Rathur SK. Impingement syndromes of the ankle. Magn Reson Imaging Clin N Am 2008;16:29–38.

35. Linklater J. MR imaging of the ankle impingement lesions. Magn Reson Imaging Clin N Am 2009;17:775–800.

36. Robinson P, White L. Soft-tissue and osseous impingement syndromes of the ankle: role of imaging in diagnosis and management. Radiographics 2002;22: 1457–71.

37. Duncan D, Mologne T, Hildebrand H, et al. The usefulness of magnetic resonance imaging in the diagnosis of anterolateral impingement of the ankle. J Foot Ankle Surg 2006;45(5):304.

38. Schaffler G, Tirman P, Stoller D, et al. Impingement syndrome of the ankle following supination external rotation trauma: MR imaging findings with arthroscopic correlation. Eur Radiol 2003;13:1357–62.

39. Rubin DA, Tishkoff NW, Britton CA, et al. Anterolateral soft-tissue impingement in the ankle: diagnosis using MR imaging. AJR Am J Roentgenol 1997;169:829–35.

40. Robinson P, White LM, Salonen DC, et al. Anterolateral ankle impingement: MR arthrographic assessment of the anterolateral recess. Radiology 2001;221(1): 186–90.

41. Farooki S, Yao L, Seeger LL. Anterolateral impingement of the ankle: effectiveness of MR imaging. Radiology 1998;207(2):357–60.

42. Jordan LK 3rd, Helms CA, Cooperman AE, et al. Magnetic resonance imaging findings in anterolateral impingement of the ankle. Skeletal Radiol 2000;29(1): 34–9.

43. Guhl JF. Soft tissue pathology. In: Guhl JF, editor. Foot and Ankle Arthroscopy. 2nd edition. Thorofare (NJ): Slack Publishing; 1993. p. 83–105.

44. Haller J, Bernt R, Seeger T, et al. MR-imaging of anterior tibiotalar impingement syndrome: agreement, sensitivity, and specificity of MR imaging and indirect MR-arthrography. Eur J Radiol 2006;58:450–60.

45. Hauger O, Moinard M, Lasalarie JS, et al. Anterolateral compartment of the ankle in the lateral impingement syndrome: appearance on CT arthrography. Radiology 1999;173:686–90.

46. Takao M, Uchio Y, Naito K, et al. Arthroscopic treatment for anterior impingement exostosis of the ankle: application of three – dimensional computed tomography. Foot Ankle Int 2004;25(2):59–62.

47. Tol J, van Dijk CN. Anterior ankle impingement. Foot Ankle Clin N Am 2006;11: 297–310.

48. DeBerardino TM, Arciero RA, Taylor DC. Arthroscopic treatment of soft-tissue impingement of the ankle in athletes. Arthroscopy 1997;13:492–8.

49. Gulish H, Sullivan R, Aronow M. Arthroscopic treatment of soft-tissue impingement lesions of the ankle in adolescents. Foot Ankle Int 2005;26(4):204.

50. Rasmussen S, Hjorth Jensen C. Arthroscopic treatment of impingement of the ankle reduces pain and enhances function. Scand J Med Sci Sports 2002;12: 69–72.

51. Hassan AH. Treatment of anterolateral impingements of the ankle joint by arthroscopy. Knee Surg Sports Traumatol Arthrosc 2007;15:1150–4.

52. Kim SH, Ha KI. Arthroscopic treatment for impingement of the anterolateral soft tissues of the ankle. J Bone Joint Surg Br 2000;82:1019–21.

53. El-Sayed A. Arthroscopic treatment of anterolateral impingement of the ankle. J Foot Ankle Surg 2010;49:219–23.

54. Edmonds E, Chanmbers R, Kaufman E, et al. Anterolateral ankle impingement in adolescents: outcomes of nonoperative and operative treatment. J Pediatr Orthop 2010;30(2):186–91.

55. Ogilvie-Harris DJ, Mahomed N, Demaziere A. Anterior impingement of the ankle treated by arthroscopic removal of bony spurs. J Bone Joint Surg Br 1993;75: 437–40.

56. Reynaert P, Gelen G, Geens G. Arthroscopic treatment of anterior impingement of the ankle. Acta Orthop Belg 1994;60(4):384–8.

57. Tol JL, Verheyen CP, van Dijk CN. Arthroscopic treatment of anterior impingement in the ankle. J Bone Joint Surg Br 2001;83(1):9–13.

58. Ferkel RD, Guhl J, Van Buecken K, et al. Complications in ankle arthroscopy: analysis of the first 518 cases. Orthop Trans 1992;16:726–7.

59. Baums MH, Kahl E, Schultz W, et al. Clinical outcome of the arthroscopic management of sports-related "anterior ankle pain": a prospective study. Knee Surg Sports Traumatol Arthrosc 2006;14:482–6.

Arthroscopic Ankle Arthrodesis

Michael S. Lee, DPM[a,b,*]

KEYWORDS

• Ankle • Arthrodesis • Arthroscopy • Fusion • Arthritis

Despite the increasing popularity of total ankle replacement (TAR), ankle arthrodesis remains the gold standard for the treatment of end-stage ankle arthritis.[1,2] Historically, open techniques have been used for ankle arthrodesis. Many variations and techniques, including transfibular, anterior, and medial approaches and miniarthrotomy, have been described.[3–17] Inherent disadvantages to these open techniques include postoperative pain, delayed union or nonunion, wound complications, shortening, prolonged healing times, and prolonged hospital stays.[18–20]

Arthroscopic ankle arthrodesis provides the foot and ankle surgeon with an alternative to the traditional open techniques. Arthroscopic ankle arthrodesis has demonstrated faster union rates, decreased complications, reduced postoperative pain, and shorter hospital stays.[3,20–29] Although once considered technically difficult, advancements in techniques and instrumentation have reduced the learning curve once encountered with the arthroscopic technique.

Schneider[30] first reported arthroscopic ankle arthrodesis in 1983, and described faster time to union, earlier mobilization, and reduced patient morbidity. Recent studies have demonstrated similar results, with faster union rates comparable with those using current open techniques, fewer complications, and shorter hospital stays.[3,21–23,29] This article discusses the indications, technique, and complications associated with arthroscopic ankle arthrodesis.

INDICATIONS/CONTRAINDICATIONS

Arthroscopic ankle arthrodesis may be indicated in patients with end-stage arthritis caused by rheumatoid arthritis, posttraumatic arthritis, arthrogryphosis, septic arthritis, inflammatory arthritis, avascular necrosis of the talus, idiopathic

Portions of this article previously appeared in Lee MS, Millward DM. Arthroscopic ankle arthrodesis. Clin Podiatr Med Surg 2009;26:273–282.
a College of Podiatric Medicine and Surgery, Des Moines University, Des Moines, IA, USA
b Foot and Ankle Surgery, Capital Orthopaedics and Sports Medicine, PC 12499 University Avenue, Suite 210, Clive, IA 50325, USA
* Foot and Ankle Surgery, Capital Orthopaedics and Sports Medicine, PC 12499 University Avenue, Suite 210, Clive, IA 50325.
E-mail address: mlee@dsmcapitalortho.com

Clin Podiatr Med Surg 28 (2011) 511–521
doi:10.1016/j.cpm.2011.04.008
0891-8422/11/$ – see front matter © 2011 Elsevier Inc. All rights reserved.

osteoarthritis, and chronic ankle instability. Posttraumatic arthritis is the most frequently encountered cause.[21]

The primary indication for ankle arthrodesis is persistent pain in the arthritic ankle joint that has not responded to conservative treatments, including analgesics, nonsteroidal antiinflammatory drugs, corticosteroid injections, and orthoses or bracing for several months.[3,22,28] Although not currently approved by the US Food and Drug Administration for the ankle joint, hyaluronase injections may also be used before proceeding with arthrodesis or replacement.

Limitations of arthroscopic ankle arthrodesis are typically related to deformity or malalignment about the ankle joint. Various studies have indicated that malalignment greater than 10° to 15° makes reduction of the ankle joint and deformity difficult.[23,31] Ferkel and Hewitt[27] indicated that patients with significant ankle deformity, either significant varus or valgus, are better suited for an open technique and those who require arthrodesis in situ are better suited for the arthroscopic technique. Tang and colleagues[32] stated that arthroscopy is not advised when a large ankle deformity is present. A study by Gougoulias and colleagues[26] showed that patients with marked deformity of greater than 10° to 15° of varus or valgus can be treated effectively using arthroscopy, depending on surgeon experience.

In addition to significant malalignment, Collman and colleagues[22] noted that contraindications of arthroscopic ankle arthrodesis include excessive bone loss, neuropathic joints, active infections, and poor bone stock. Avascular necrosis of the talus may also be a contraindication.

SURGICAL TECHNIQUE

Arthroscopic ankle arthrodesis is performed under general or spinal anesthesia. A thigh tourniquet is typically used for hemostasis, and the leg is prepped to the tibial tuberosity. A bump under the ipsilateral hip is used to slightly rotate the leg internally.

The ankle is insufflated with approximately 20 mL of normal sterile saline using an 18-gauge needle. Standard anteromedial and anterolateral portals are used. A 2.7-mm 30° arthroscope is then introduced into the ankle joint. The author prefers to use large joint power shavers and burrs while using a 2.7-mm arthroscope rather than the 4.0-mm arthroscope. A noninvasive ankle distractor is applied to the ankle to allow for complete visualization from anterior to posterior, as well as both the medial and lateral gutters (**Fig. 1**).

A 3.85-mm full-radius incisor blade is used to aggressively debride the anterior joint of any hypertrophic synovium, fibrosis, or loose bodies. In some cases, aggressive resection of anterior tibiotalar osteophytes is required for proper joint visualization. A curette is inserted to aggressively remove any remaining articular cartilage (**Fig. 2**). A grasping forceps or resector may be used to remove the cartilage fragments that typically collect in the posterior aspect of the joint (**Fig. 3**). A 4.0-mm full-radius burr or 4.85-mm acromion burr is then used to resect the subchondral plate (**Fig. 4**). A curved osteotome is then used to fish scale the subchondral plates of both the tibia and talus (**Fig. 5**). Ideally, healthy bleeding bone is visualized throughout the tibiotalar articulation (**Fig. 6**). The joint is then irrigated, and all loose bodies or fragments are evacuated.

All arthroscopic instrumentation is then removed from the ankle joint. Platelet-rich plasma or other bone graft substitutes may then be inserted into the ankle joint at the surgeon's discretion. The noninvasive distractor is removed from the foot. Proper bony apposition is confirmed using fluoroscopy. Care is also taken to confirm proper positioning clinically.

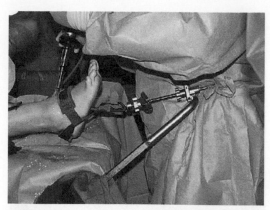

Fig. 1. Noninvasive ankle distractor is used for joint visualization. (*From* Lee MS, Millward DM. Arthroscopic ankle arthrodesis. Clin Podiatr Med Surg 2009;26:274; with permission.)

Fixation is achieved with 2 or 3 large-diameter cannulated screws. Typically, one screw is placed from the lateral talar process into the medial tibia, the second from the posterior tibia into the talar neck, and the third (if desired) from the lateral tibia into the posteromedial talus (**Fig. 7**).

The portals and stab incisions for screw placement are closed with simple sutures. The extremity is placed in a controlled ankle motion (CAM) boot. In most cases, the patient is discharged on the day of surgery. Sutures are removed 1 week postoperatively, and a below-the-knee cast is applied. Strict adherence to non–weight bearing is followed for 6 to 7 weeks. Weight bearing is then advanced based on radiographic healing and clinical symptoms in the CAM boot (**Fig. 8**). Typically, at approximately 10 weeks postoperatively, the patient's foot is placed in a rocker-bottom sole shoe and ankle-foot orthosis (AFO), and activities are advanced as tolerated. The AFO is continued for up to an additional 3 months, and the rocker-bottom sole is continued according to the patient's preference.

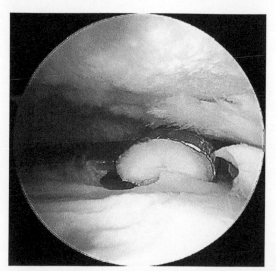

Fig. 2. Curettage of the remaining articular surface. (*From* Lee MS, Millward DM. Arthroscopic ankle arthrodesis. Clin Podiatr Med Surg 2009;26:275; with permission.)

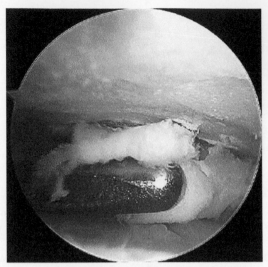

Fig. 3. Removal of the cartilage fragments after aggressive curettage. (*From* Lee MS, Millward DM. Arthroscopic ankle arthrodesis. Clin Podiatr Med Surg 2009;26:276; with permission.)

DISCUSSION

Arthroscopic ankle arthrodesis has been well studied and has demonstrated favorable postoperative outcomes.[20–29] Advantages include decreased time to union, diminished postoperative pain, comparable union rates, shorter hospital stays, and earlier patient mobilization.[20–29,33–36] Preservation of the bony contour and the large amount of cancellous bony contact allows for significant stability and rigid internal fixation.[22,36] This outcome is contradictory to the traditional open techniques, which have often implemented planal resection, decreasing bony contact and inherent stability. In

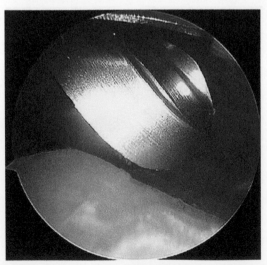

Fig. 4. Full-radius burr is used to resect the subchondral plate. (*From* Lee MS, Millward DM. Arthroscopic ankle arthrodesis. Clin Podiatr Med Surg 2009;26:276; with permission.)

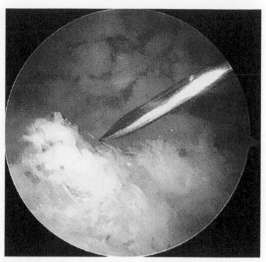

Fig. 5. Fish scaling the talus with a curved osteotome in preparation for arthrodesis. (*From* Lee MS, Millward DM. Arthroscopic ankle arthrodesis. Clin Podiatr Med Surg 2009;26: 277; with permission.)

addition, flat-topping the talus and tibia makes proper positioning of the foot in the sagittal plane significantly more difficult because precise bone cuts are required. O'Brien and colleagues[20] showed that there was a greater variability of ankle positions in patients who received the open ankle fusion compared with those who received the arthroscopic technique.

Stetson and Ferkel[31] recommended an open technique in ankles that have malrotation or anteroposterior translation of the tibiotalar joint. The investigators also believed ankles that had a deformity of greater than 15° of varus or valgus should be treated with an open technique.[31] Gougoulias and colleagues,[26] however, achieved successful

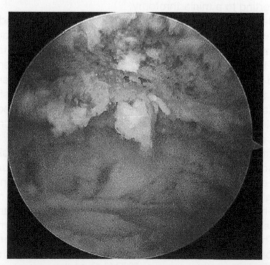

Fig. 6. Joint surfaces after preparation for arthrodesis. (*From* Lee MS, Millward DM. Arthroscopic ankle arthrodesis. Clin Podiatr Med Surg 2009;26:277; with permission.)

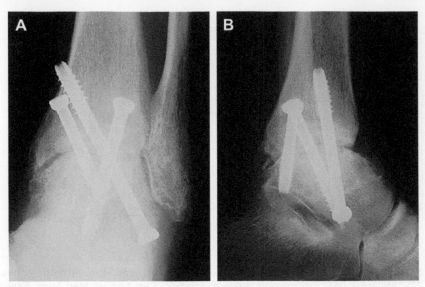

Fig. 7. Typical fixation ([A] anteroposterior view, [B] lateral view) after arthroscopic ankle arthrodesis. (*From* Lee MS, Millward DM. Arthroscopic ankle arthrodesis. Clin Podiatr Med Surg 2009;26:278; with permission.)

arthroscopic ankle arthrodeses on ankle deformities of 15° to 45° varus or valgus. The investigators point out that although they were able to successfully fuse ankles with marked deformity, there is a significant learning curve associated with the procedure.[26] Another recent study also suggests that it may be possible to fuse ankles with deformities of 25° or greater arthroscopically.[23] This author has found that malalignment up to 15° is acceptable for arthroscopic arthrodesis. In some cases, particularly in severe valgus malalignment of the ankle, the joint may be reducible clinically. In these cases, arthroscopic ankle arthrodesis is possible but preoperative planning includes the possibility of converting to a miniarthrotomy.

Union may be described in 2 different ways: clinical union and radiographic union. Clinical union is described as having a stable painless ankle joint. Radiographic union is defined as having bridging trabeculae between the tibia and the talus.[26,37]

Nonunion rates between arthroscopic ankle arthrodesis and open techniques are similar. Crosby and colleagues[38] reported a clinical fusion rate of 93% and a radiographic union rate of 74%, indicating a subset of arthroscopic ankle arthrodesis cases that have a clinical union rate of 87.2%. A nonunion rate of 7.6% was reported by Winson and colleagues[23] in their review of 118 arthroscopic ankle fusions. Similar union rates in other studies have been reported, with a range from 73% to 100%.[3,17,20,27–29,33,35,38–40]

Studies demonstrating union rates correlated with patient comorbidities have been limited primarily to rheumatoid arthritis.[39,41,42] Other variables such as history of smoking, arthritis etiology, effects of bone graft substitutes, body mass index (BMI, calculated as weight in kilograms divided by the square of height in meters), and pre-existing deformity have not been extensively studied with regard to arthroscopic ankle arthrodesis. In one study, nonunions were reported in 4 of 5 patients with posttraumatic arthritis.[22] The higher concentration of sclerotic bone adjacent to the subchondral plate may contribute to this increased incidence of nonunion, reinforcing the importance of aggressive joint resection.[29,33,41,43] Malalignment of the ankle may also predispose to nonunion of the arthroscopic ankle arthrodesis.[22]

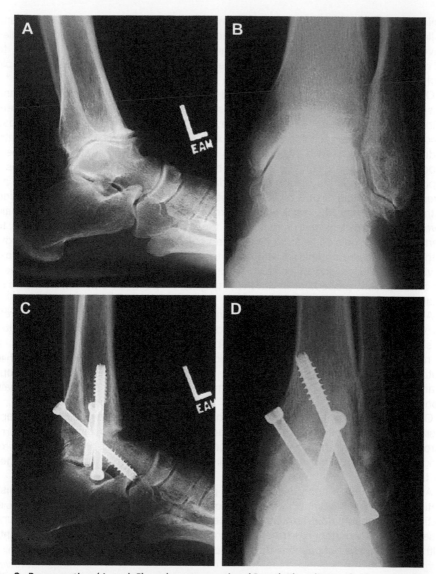

Fig. 8. Preoperative (*A* and *B*) and postoperative (*C* and *D*) radiographs for arthroscopic ankle arthrodesis. (*From* Lee MS, Millward DM. Arthroscopic ankle arthrodesis. Clin Podiatr Med Surg 2009;26:279; with permission.)

Cigarette smoking and its negative effects on both soft tissue and bone healing has been well documented.[44–49] The role of nicotine in ankle arthrodesis nonunions has also been well documented, and smoking may present a relative risk of nonunion 4 times than that seen in nonsmokers.[18,50] Collman and colleagues[22] did not see this same trend in their series of arthroscopic ankle fusions and theorized that the ill effects of smoking are countered by the minimally invasive approach.

A clear advantage to the use of arthroscopic arthrodesis over open techniques is the reduced time to fusion. Open ankle fusions have a reported average fusion time of approximately 14 weeks.[33,34] In a study of 39 arthroscopic arthrodeses, Collman and colleagues[22] reported an average fusion time of 47 days, whereas Glick and colleagues[35] noted an average fusion time of 9 weeks in 34 ankles. Other studies have noted the time to fusion for arthroscopic ankle arthrodesis from 8.9 to 12 weeks.[3,23,29] One theory to support the decreased fusion time is that the arthroscopic technique does not disrupt the periarticular blood supply facilitating healing.[29,33,35,41]

O'Brien and colleagues[20] demonstrated that the tourniquet time, blood loss, and hospitalization times were all decreased using arthroscopy. Patients who underwent arthroscopic arthrodesis had hospital stays of 1.6 days versus 3.4 days in those who underwent open techniques.[20] Use of the arthroscopic technique may greatly reduce the postoperative hospitalization period. Ogilvie-Harris and colleagues[28] reported an average discharge from the hospital of 1 day. Dent and colleagues[25] reported an average stay of less than 2 days. Zvijac and colleagues[29] reported an average hospitalization of 3 days for those who had an open procedure compared with 1 day for those who received an arthroscopic arthrodesis. They noted that pain levels were much less than expected in the arthroscopic group, leading them to perform arthroscopic ankle arthrodesis on an outpatient basis.[29] In yet another study, arthroscopic fusion compared with open techniques demonstrated significant cost savings.[51] Cameron and Ulrich[3] also reported doing arthroscopic ankle arthrodesis as an outpatient procedure. In another study of 39 patients, only 3 were not discharged on the day of the procedure.[22]

Arthroscopic ankle arthrodesis has demonstrated reduced pain postoperatively as well as lesser reliance on pain medication.[25,28,29] The author has also noted a significant decrease in postoperative pain with the arthroscopic technique. It is now common practice for arthroscopic ankle arthrodeses to be performed in outpatient surgery centers, and, generally, the decision to admit a patient postoperatively is based on comorbid deformities and not on postoperative pain concerns.

Other advantages of arthroscopic arthrodesis include decreased blood loss, less disruption of the soft tissue structures around the ankle, and diminished risk of thrombosis due to shorter immobilization times. There is also minimal loss of length of the lower limb as well as minimal clinical deformity or shape changes to the ankle.[25]

Arthroscopic ankle arthrodesis may be preferred to an open technique in at-risk patients.[22] The earlier mobilization due to a shorter time to union is beneficial in patients with rheumatoid arthritis, advanced age, diabetes, and other autoimmune diseases.[33,40] The author has used the arthroscopic technique in these at-risk patients with great success but cautions its use in patients with peripheral neuropathy.

SUMMARY

Arthroscopic ankle arthrodesis provides the foot and ankle surgeon with an alternative to traditional open techniques. Advancements in arthroscopic techniques and instrumentation have made the procedure easier to perform. Arthroscopic ankle arthrodesis has demonstrated faster rates of union, decreased complications, reduced postoperative pain, and shorter hospital stays.[3,20–29] Adherence to sound surgical techniques, particularly with regard to joint preparation, is critical for success. Comorbidities, such as increased BMI, history of smoking, malalignment, and posttraumatic arthritis, should be carefully considered when contemplating arthroscopic ankle arthrodesis. Although TAR continues to grow in popularity, arthroscopic ankle arthrodesis remains a viable alternative for management of the end-stage arthritic ankle.

REFERENCES

1. Coester LM, Saltman CL, Leapold J, et al. Long-term results following ankle arthrodesis for post-traumatic arthritis. J Bone Joint Surg 2001;83:219–28.
2. Buck P, Morrey BF, Chao EY. The optimum position of arthrodesis of the ankle. J Bone Joint Surg 1987;69:1052–62.
3. Cameron SE, Ulrich P. Arthroscopic arthrodesis of the ankle joint. Arthroscopy 2000;16:21–6.
4. Cheng YM, Chen SK, Chen JC, et al. Revision of ankle arthrodesis. Foot Ankle Int 2003;24:321–5.
5. Colgrove RC, Bruffey JD. Ankle arthrodesis: combined internal-external fixation. Foot Ankle Int 2001;22:92–7.
6. Adams JC. Arthrodesis of the ankle joint: experiences with transfibular approach. J Bone Joint Surg 1948;30(B):506–11.
7. Frankel JP, Bacardi BE. Chevron ankle arthrodesis with bone grafting and internal fixation. J Foot Surg 1986;25:234–40.
8. Anderson R. Concentric arthrodesis of the ankle joint: a transmalleolar approach. J Bone Joint Surg 1945;27:37–48.
9. Baciu CC. A simple technique for arthrodesis of the ankle. J Bone Joint Surg 1986;68(B):266–7.
10. Campbell P. Arthrodesis of the ankle with modified distraction-compression and bone-grafting. J Bone Joint Surg 1990;72:552–6.
11. Campbell CJ, Rinehart WT, Kalenak A. Arthrodesis of the ankle: deep autogenous inlay grafts with maximum cancellous bone apposition. J Bone Joint Surg 1974; 56:63–70.
12. Vogler HW. Ankle fusion: techniques and complications. J Foot Surg 1991;30:80–4.
13. Thordarson DB, Markolf KL, Cracchiolo A. Arthrodesis of the ankle with cancellous-bone screws and fibular strut graft. Biomechanical analysis. J Bone Joint Surg 1990;72:1359–63.
14. Mauerer RC, Cimino WR, Cox CV, et al. Transarticular cross-screw fixation; a technique of ankle arthrodesis. Clin Orthop 1991;268:56–69.
15. Morgan CD, Henke JA, Bailey RW, et al. Long-term results of tibiotalar arthrodesis. J Bone Joint Surg 1985;67:546–50.
16. Mears DC, Gordon RG, Kann SE, et al. Ankle arthrodesis with an anterior tension plate. Clin Orthop 1991;268:70–7.
17. Paremain GD, Miller SD, Myerson MS. Ankle arthrodesis: results after the miniarthrotomy technique. Foot Ankle Int 1996;17:247–51.
18. Frey C, Halikus NM, Vu-Rose T, et al. A review of ankle arthrodesis: predisposing factors to nonunion. Foot Ankle Int 1994;15(11):581–4.
19. Morrey BF, Wiedeman GP Jr. Complications and long-term results of ankle arthrodeses following trauma. J Bone Joint Surg Am 1980;62(5):777–84.
20. O'Brien TS, Hart TS, Shereff MJ, et al. Open versus arthroscopic ankle arthrodesis: a comparative study. Foot Ankle Int 1999;20(6):368–74.
21. Stone JW. Arthroscopic ankle arthrodesis. Foot Ankle Clin 2006;11(2):361–8.
22. Collman DR, Kaas MH, Schuberth JM. Arthroscopic ankle arthrodesis: factors influencing union in 39 consecutive patients. Foot Ankle Int 2006;27:1079–85.
23. Winson IG, Robinson DE, Allen PE. Arthroscopic ankle arthrodesis. J Bone Joint Surg Br 2005;87(3):343–7.
24. Kats J, van Kampen A, de Waal-Malefijt MC. Improvement in technique for arthroscopic ankle fusion: results in 15 patients. Knee Surg Sports Traumatol Arthrosc 2003;11(1):46–9.

25. Dent CM, Patil M, Fairclough JA. Arthroscopic ankle arthrodesis. J Bone Joint Surg Br 1993;75(5):830–2.

26. Gougoulias NE, Agathangelidis FG, Parsons SW. Arthroscopic ankle arthrodesis. Foot Ankle Int 2007;28(6):695–706.

27. Ferkel RD, Hewitt M. Long-term results of arthroscopic ankle arthrodesis. Foot Ankle Int 2005;26(4):275–80.

28. Ogilvie-Harris DJ, Lieberman I, Fitsialos D. Arthroscopically assisted arthrodesis for osteoarthrotic ankles. J Bone Joint Surg Am 1993;75(8):1167–74.

29. Zvijac JE, Lemak L, Schurhoff MR, et al. Analysis of arthroscopically assisted ankle arthrodesis. Arthroscopy 2002;18(1):70–5.

30. Schneider D. Arthroscopic ankle fusion. Arthroscopic Video J 1983;3.

31. Stetson WB, Ferkel RD. Ankle arthroscopy: II. Indications and results. J Am Acad Orthop Surg 1996;4(1):24–34.

32. Tang KL, Li QH, Chen GX, et al. Arthroscopically assisted ankle fusion in patients with end-stage tuberculosis. Arthroscopy 2007;23(9):919–22.

33. Myerson MS, Quill G. Ankle arthrodesis. A comparison of an arthroscopic and an open method of treatment. Clin Orthop Relat Res 1991;(268):84–95.

34. Mann RA, Van Manen JW, Wapner K, et al. Ankle fusion. Clin Orthop Relat Res 1991;268:49–55.

35. Glick JM, Morgan CD, Myerson MS, et al. Ankle arthrodesis using an arthroscopic method: long-term follow-up of 34 cases. Arthroscopy 1996;12(4):428–34.

36. Jay RM. A new concept of ankle arthrodesis via arthroscopic technique. Clin Podiatr Med Surg 2000;17(1):147–57.

37. Monroe MT, Beals TC, Manoli A 2nd. Clinical outcome of arthrodesis of the ankle using rigid internal fixation with cancellous screws. Foot Ankle Int 1999;20(4): 227–31.

38. Crosby LA, Yee TC, Formanek TS, et al. Complications following arthroscopic ankle arthrodesis. Foot Ankle Int 1996;17:340–2.

39. Corso SJ, Zimmer TJ. Technique and clinical evaluation of arthroscopic ankle arthrodesis. Arthroscopy 1995;11:585–90.

40. Jerosch J, Steinbeck J, Schroder M, et al. Arthroscopically assisted arthrodesis of the ankle joint. Arch Orthop Trauma Surg 1996;115:182–9.

41. DeVriese L, Dereymaeker G, Fabry G. Arthroscopic ankle arthrodesis preliminary report. Acta Orthop Belg 1994;60:389–92.

42. Turan I, Wredmark T, Fellander-Tsai L. Arthroscopic ankle arthrodesis in rheumatoid arthritis. Clin Orthop 1995;320:110–4.

43. Blair HC. Comminuted fractures and fracture-dislocations of the body of the astragalus: operative treatment. Am J Surg 1943;59:37–43.

44. Brown CW, Orme TJ, Richardson HD. The rate of pseudoarthrosis (surgical nonunion) in patients who are smokers and patients who are nonsmokers; a comparison study. Spine 1986;11:942–3.

45. Glasman SD, Anagnost SC, Parker A, et al. The effect of cigarette smoking and smoking cessation on spinal fusion. Spine 2000;25:2608–15.

46. Haverstock BD, Mandracchia VJ. Cigarette smoking and bone healing: implication in foot and ankle surgery. J Foot Ankle Surg 1998;37:69–74.

47. Ishikawa SN, Murphy GA, Richardson EG. The effect of cigarette smoking on hindfoot fusions. Foot Ankle Int 2002;23:996–8.

48. Nolan J, Jenkins RA, Kurihara K, et al. The acute effects of cigarette smoke exposure on experimental skin flaps. Plast Reconst Surg 1985;75:544–51.

49. Sherwin MA, Gastwirth CM. Detrimental effects of cigarette smoking on lower extremity wound healing. J Foot Surg 1990;29:84–7.

50. Cobb TK, Gabrielsen TA, Campbell DC 2nd, et al. Cigarette smoking and nonunion after ankle arthrodesis. Foot Ankle 1994;15:64–7.
51. Petersen KS, Lee MS, Buddecke DE. Arthroscopic versus open ankle arthrodesis: a retrospective cost analysis. J Foot Ankle Surg 2010;49:242–7.

Arthroscopically Assisted Treatment of Ankle Injuries

George Gumann, DPM[a],*,[1], Graham A. Hamilton, DPM[b,c,1]

KEYWORDS

• Ankle injuries • Arthroscopy • Ankle fractures
• Intra-articular fractures

Ankle fractures that are displaced and unstable have traditionally required surgical intervention to obtain an anatomic reduction and stabilization with internal fixation (open reduction and internal fixation [ORIF]).[1,2] This necessitates a surgical exposure of adequate size to visualize and reduce the fracture fragments as well as allow the delivery of appropriate fixation. The repair also requires inspection of the ankle articular surfaces for any damage. Chondral and osteochondral fragments, if identified, should be addressed with excision or repair. There is a biologic price for this strategy. Open techniques usually require extensive soft tissue dissection that can potentially compromise the blood supply to the osseous structures and affect healing. Arthroscopy is an expedient tool in the management of intra-articular fractures of the ankle. It can provide the surgeon with the ability to help anatomically reduce a fracture under direct visualization and sometimes be combined with a minimally invasive ORIF. It also affords the surgeon the ability to address any articular injury with minimal biologic risk.[3,4]

Indications: fractures amenable to arthroscopic assistance using either a traditional open or a minimally invasive approach.

1. Unimalleolar fractures
   a. Weber Type A fibular fracture
   b. Fractures of the medial malleolus
2. Certain minimally displaced bimalleolar or trimalleolar fractures

---

[a] Department of Surgery, Orthopedic Clinic, Martin Army Community Hospital, 7950 Martin Loop, Fort Benning, GA 31905-5637, USA
[b] Department of Orthopedics, The Permanente Medical Group Inc, 4501 Sand Creek Road, Antioch, CA 94531, USA
[c] Department of Podiatric Surgery, Kaiser Permanente, Antioch, CA, USA
[1] The opinions of the authors should not be construed as reflecting official policy of the U.S. Army Medical Department.
* Corresponding author.
E-mail address: g.gumann@mchsi.com

Clin Podiatr Med Surg 28 (2011) 523–538
doi:10.1016/j.cpm.2011.04.002
0891-8422/11/$ – see front matter. Published by Elsevier Inc.

podiatric.theclinics.com

3. Bimalleolar equivalent fracture
4. Fractures of the proximal fibula (Maissoneuve fracture)
5. Unstable diastasis
6. Tillaux fracture
7. Triplane fracture
8. Selected pilon fractures
9. Talus fracture
10. Acute osteochondral fractures of the talus.

Contraindications: to using arthroscopic assistance

1. A grossly compromised soft tissue envelope
2. Fracture that is significantly displaced that obviously demands ORIF
3. Medically unstable patient.

SURGICAL ASSESSMENT

The patient initially requires a thorough physical examination coupled with appropriate radiographic evaluation of the ankle along with the leg or foot as indicated. With the patient hemodynamically stable, immobilization of the fracture is performed along with a closed reduction if necessary to relocate a subluxation or dislocation. A compressive dressing and splint/fracture brace is applied. Initial surgery performed within 6 hours of injury is ideal. If the surgery is delayed, then the timing of the procedure will depend on the recovery of the soft tissue to decrease the likelihood of postoperative wound problems.[5] This principle of allowing the soft tissue to "settle" must be respected. For unusual adult fracture patterns and more routinely in specific pediatric ankle fractures, a computed tomography (CT) scan is required to fully observe the fracture configuration and aid with developing an approach to deliver fixation. The question then becomes which fractures may benefit from arthroscopic assistance, and also, which fractures can be successfully managed from a minimally invasive approach.

PEARLS IN ARTHROSCOPIC TECHNIQUE

Large (4.0 mm) and small joint (2.7 mm) arthroscopes can be used depending on the size of the patient. Most fracture patterns can be visualized with the standard anteromedial and anterolateral portals. Occasionally, an accessory portal is necessary to aid in reduction or for an alternate view of the fracture. Gravity inflow is preferred, avoiding arthroscopic pumps that can increase inflow pressure resulting in fluid extravasation. Extravasation of the ingress fluid from the arthroscopic procedure can increase the risk of wound problems or compartment syndrome. It can also cause the soft tissue envelope to swell, making it difficult to palpate osseous structures for a minimally invasive ORIF. Two bags with 3 L of lactated Ringers solution is suspended 3 to 4 feet above the operating table. Inflow through the cannula and a separate portal for outflow aids with distention and visualization. Another problem can be the disruption of the capsule and ligaments that prevents distention by allowing fluid escape, limiting the ability to see. Generally with most injury patterns, the joint can be entered without any distraction, as an unstable mortise allows for easier passage of instruments. Distraction is occasionally needed to help gain access to the ankle joint (**Fig. 1**).[6] It can be helpful in visualizing the posterior aspect of the ankle joint or examining the inferior tibial plafond. Upon entering the joint, one encounters varying degrees of hemarthrosis, synovium, and joint debris. This requires

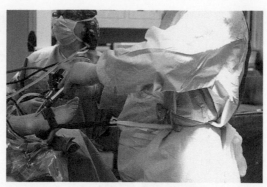

Fig. 1. Modified ankle distractor technique using noninvasive ankle strap (Smith-Nephew) and a kerlex roll.

evacuation by joint lavage and the introduction of a synovial shaver. With joint debridement, the fracture will be visible. The fracture site can be debrided of hematoma and any entrapped periosteum with a dental pick. Certain fractures can now be reduced percutaneously with a pointed reduction forceps. The reduction is checked with arthroscopic and fluoroscopic control. If anatomically reduced, then internal fixation can be delivered.

TREATMENT OF SPECIFIC FRACTURES
Pediatric Ankle Fractures

Nearly 40% of physeal injuries in children are ankle fractures and more than half of these occur in sports.[7] With pediatric ankle fractures, the transitional fractures of Tillaux and the triplane fracture are amenable to athroscopically assisted percutaneous techniques. The Tillaux fracture is a Salter-Harris Type III fracture (**Fig. 2**).[8] It is seen in the older adolescent, as it is the last part of the distal tibia epiphyseal plate to fuse. It usually occurs within a year of complete closure of the distal tibial physis. The injury mechanism is external rotation that produces a quadrilateral-shaped fracture fragment on the anterolateral aspect of the tibia. This fragment is displaced and rotated laterally with a gap separating the fragments but normally without step-off. A CT scan best demonstrates this fracture. An arthroscopic approach can easily visualize the fracture along the anterior aspect of the tibia and allow for debridement of the hematoma. A percutaneously placed pointed reduction forceps can reduce the fracture under arthroscopic and fluoroscopic visualization. A cannulated lag screw can then be delivered percutaneously under fluoroscopic control. The screw can be perpendicular to the ankle joint or angled slightly superiorly. Crossing the epiphyseal plate with a screw is not an issue, as this is the last portion of the physis to close.

The tibial triplane fracture is a complex injury defined by sagittal, transverse, and coronal components. The triplane mechanism of injury is external rotation along with pronation and plantarflexion (**Fig. 3**).[7,9–12] It is seen in children slightly younger than for the Tillaux fracture. It is classically described as a combination Salter-Harris Type II in the metaphysis and Type III fracture in the epiphysis. It extends from the ankle joint across the epiphysis through the epiphyseal plate progressing into the metaphysis. Perhaps, it should best be thought of as a variation Type IV fracture. This fracture requires a CT scan for evaluation and usually has 2 or 3 parts, although

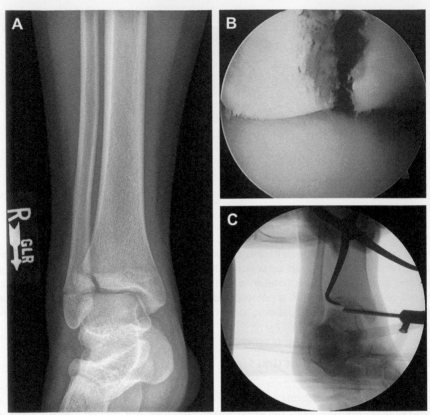

Fig. 2. (A) A 12-year-old girl sustained a Tillaux fracture playing basketball. (B) Arthroscopic picture demonstrating fracture. (C) Fluoroscopic imaging during reduction. (D) Intraoperative photograph demonstrating fracture reduction and fixation with arthroscopic guidance. (E) Fluoroscopic view of reduction and fixation. (F) Arthroscopic view of reduction (G) Fluoroscopic view of reduction and internal screw fixation.

4 parts have been reported.[11] Operative treatment is recommended if the displacement is 2 mm or more.[9–12] The degree of displacement can vary greatly in these injuries. If the displacement is not too large, then the triplane fracture can be approached as described for the Tillaux fracture with arthroscopically assisted percutaneous reduction and internal fixation. Arthroscopic visualization of the fracture line anteriorly along the tibia is usually good. One or 2 lag screws are placed in the epiphysis depending on the number of fragments, followed by 1 or 2 screws in the metaphyseal component. If the displacement is large, then a closed reduction will be necessary to bring the fracture fragments into closer apposition. Then an arthroscopically assisted percutaneous method can be used. Entrapped periosteum can thwart this approach and will then require ORIF.

Adult Ankle Fractures

In adult ankle fractures, arthroscopically assisted minimally invasive techniques can sometimes be used. Unimalleolar fractures that are not significantly displaced are the best for application of this method. On occasion, mildly displaced bimalleolar

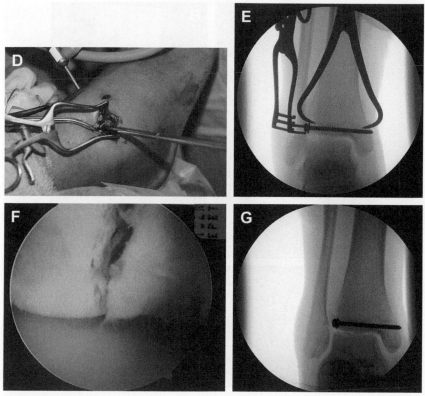

Fig. 2. (*continued*)

and trimalleolar fractures can be successfully managed in this way. Of the unimalleolar fractures, the best candidates are the transverse fracture of the lateral malleolus and the obliquely or vertically oriented fracture of the medial malleolus.

The isolated transverse fracture of the lateral malleolus below the level of the syndesmosis (Weber A) is usually not displaced significantly. It is typically gapped and/or slightly displaced laterally. It is easily identified arthroscopically and percutaneously reduced (**Fig. 4**). The fracture can be reduced with manual pressure externally or with a probe intra-articularly. Many times, the fracture can be manipulated with pointed reduction forceps percutaneously. Once reduced, a cannulated intramedullary lag screw can be delivered from the tip of the lateral malleolus in a cephalad direction. An isolated obliquely or vertically oriented fracture of the medial malleolus can be reduced and fixated with this technique. This is because the fracture pattern allows better access and direction for reduction forceps placement. The fracture is arthroscopically visualized anteromedially at the bend of the tibia. Once reduction is accomplished, fixation is usually achieved with 2 cannulated lag screws. For a vertically oriented medial malleolar fracture, an additional fixation option is a percutaneously placed plate for an antiglide function. In certain scenarios, periosteal interposition can prevent reduction and require formal ORIF. Sometimes, a small incision at the apex of the fracture can aid in reduction and evaluation of the reduction. Care must be exercised, as many vertically oriented medial malleolar fractures have

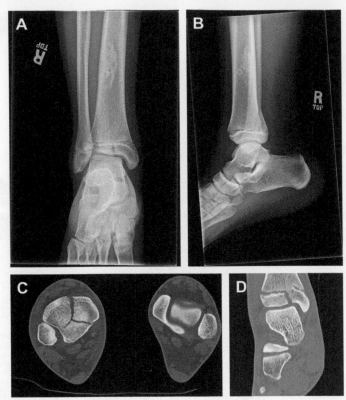

Fig. 3. (*A*) Anteroposterior (AP) and (*B*) lateral views of a 15-year-old boy who sustained a triplane fracture in a high school football game. (*C–E*) CT scan views of 3-part triplane fracture. (*F*) Arthroscopic view of fracture displacement. (*G*) Arthroscopic view of reduction. (*H*) Mortise and (*I*) lateral views demonstrate anatomic reduction and good position of the screws.

osteochondral fragments or sometimes an impacted tibial plafond, which requires traditional ORIF. The transverse fracture of the medial malleolus has been somewhat more resistant to the arthroscopically assisted percutaneous strategy because it commonly has periosteal entrapment within the fracture and the transverse configuration makes it more difficult to place a reduction forceps (**Fig. 5**).

Minimally displaced bimalleolar or trimalleolar fractures on occasion can be treated with arthroscopically assisted minimally invasive means. This is especially true if either the medial malleolus or the fibula fracture are minimally displaced or nondisplaced. It is acceptable to fixate one side in a minimally invasive fashion and the other with traditional ORIF. Arthroscopic evaluation can aid in any reduction and in identifying osteochondral damage. The arthroscope can be inserted at the beginning of the procedure through traditional portals or it can be placed through an open arthrotomy incision.

Arthroscopic assistance is more commonly successful when used with the bimalleolar equivalent fracture (**Fig. 6**). This is a fracture of the fibula along with a ruptured deltoid ligament. The arthroscope is placed to evaluate the ankle joint for osteochondral defects, especially those on the medial talar dome. Ferkel and colleagues[3] reported that approximately 80% of ankle fractures have a chondral or osteochondral

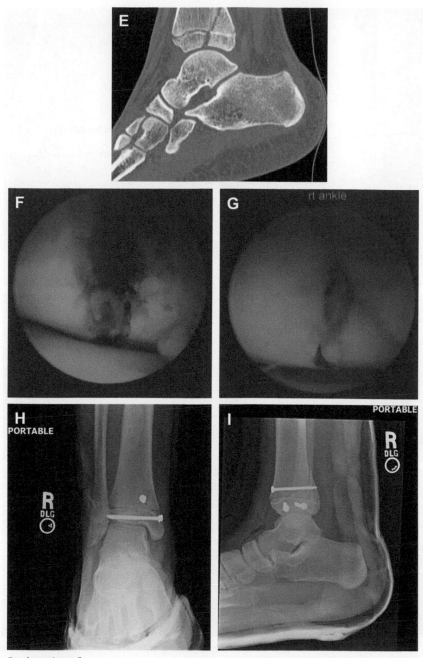

Fig. 3. (continued)

lesion. Leontaritis and colleagues[4] noted in 283 ankle fractures that underwent ORIF along with ankle arthroscopy that 73% were observed to have chondral defects. The articular damage can range from impactions and excoriations to chondral or osteo-chondral fragments. There is no treatment for impactions or excoriations; however,

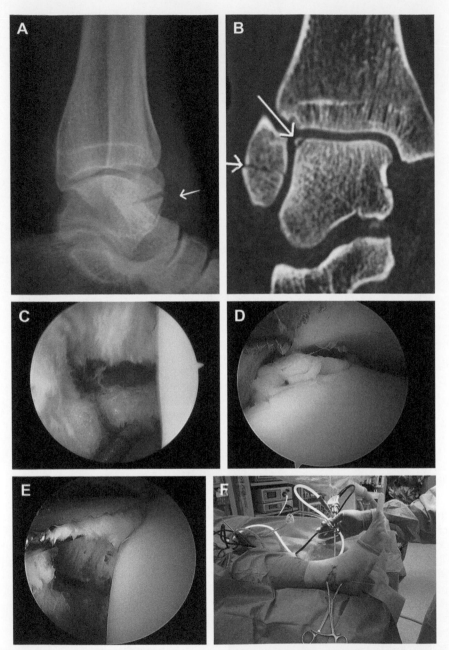

Fig. 4. (*A*) Lateral view of Weber A fracture involving the lateral malleolus. (*B*) CT scan demonstrating lateral malleolus fracture and lateral talar dome osteochondral fracture. (*C*) Arthroscopic view of fibular fracture. (*D*) Arthroscopic view of acute lateral talar dome osteochondral fracture. (*E*) Osteochondral fracture is being excised and the fracture of the lateral malleolus can also be visualized. (*F*) Percutaneous fibular reduction under arthroscopic control. (*G*) Fluoroscopic view of fracture reduction and provisional stabilization. (*H*) Arthroscopic view of reduction. (*I*) Mortise radiograph of anatomically reduced fibular fracture fixated with a cancellous lag screw and excision of osteochondral fracture.

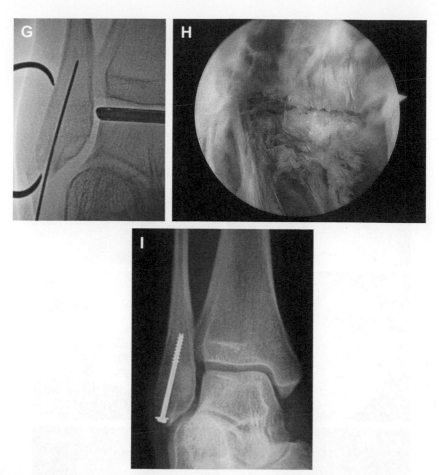

Fig. 4. (*continued*)

they can be documented and used to assess the prognosis. If a fragment needs excision, it can be done arthroscopically or through an arthrotomy. If the articular surface is undamaged, then the medial side does not need to be surgically exposed. The deltoid ligament does not require primary repair as long as the fibular fracture is anatomically reduced, fixated, and the syndesmosis is stable.[13] The fibula can now be anatomically reduced and fixed using traditional ORIF. However, occasionally the fibula in a Weber B or a low Weber C fracture can be approached with a percutaneous or minimally invasive approach. Using fluoroscopic control, the fibular fracture is percutaneously reduced with a reduction forceps. The distal fragment is described as spiral or spiral-oblique and needs to be manipulated to gain length and internally rotated. This is not necessarily easy. If successful, a percutaneous lag screw is placed from anterior to posterior inclined slightly inferiorly to make it perpendicular to the fracture. There is always concern for the possibility of iatrogenic damage to the superficial peroneal nerve. A small incision is placed at the inferior aspect of the lateral malleolus and an extraperiosteal soft tissue tunnel developed. A one-third tubular plate (locking or nonlocking) is contoured and then directed through the incision in a superior direction. It is positioned with fluoroscopic control and fixated to the fibula. The screws in

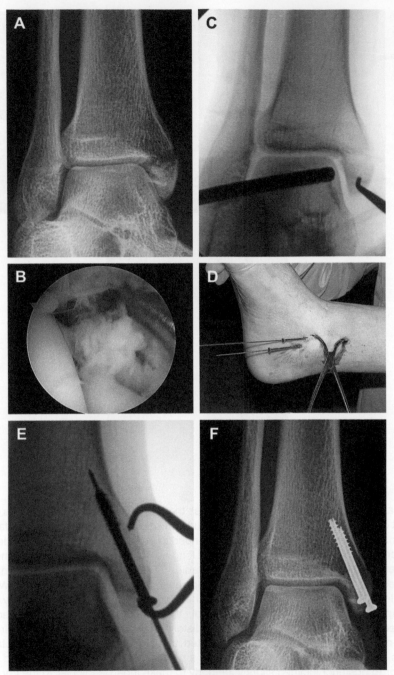

Fig. 5. (*A*) AP radiograph demonstrates transverse fracture of the medial malleolus. (*B*) Arthroscopic view of fracture. (*C*) Fluoroscopic view of fracture manipulation. (*D*) Clinical photograph of percutaneous reduction and internal fixation. (*E*) Fluoroscopic view. (*F*) Intra-operative radiograph demonstrating anatomic reduction and good position screws.

the distal holes over the lateral malleolus can be placed directly through the incision. The proximal screws can be placed percutaneously. In a low Weber C fracture, another option is to place a small incision just at the fracture site to reduce it and possibly place a lag screw. From this small incision, an extraperiosteal tunnel is developed superiorly and inferiorly. The plate can be manipulated through this incision or a minimally invasive incision can be made more inferiorly and the plate slid proximately. The problem is the more proximal the plate is placed, the more likely it will be covered by the peroneal muscles and the harder it will be to manipulate the plate and deliver screws percutaneously. Sometimes, a small incision is needed over the proximal aspect of the plate. However, the inability to reduce a fracture will lead to abandoning the minimally invasive approach and proceeding to formal ORIF. This can be caused by soft tissue entrapment, inability to actually manipulate the fracture fragments, osseous impaction, difficulty in placing internal fixation, or difficulty in interpreting the fluoroscopic images.

Another injury pattern that is well served using arthroscopic assistance is the Maisonneuve fracture.[14] This is because the proximal fibular fracture many times is nondisplaced or minimally displaced. Because it is fixated in an indirect manner, the ankle can be arthroscopically evaluated, the syndesmosis provisionally stabilized with a large pointed reduction forceps, and the transyndesmotic screws delivered percutaneously with fluoroscopic visualization. An unstable syndesmotic (high ankle sprain) injury can also be managed in the same manner (**Fig. 7**).[15]

High-energy pilon fractures are now generally treated in a 2-stage approach.[16–19] The first stage is application of an external fixator with or without fibular reduction and fixation. The second stage is removal of the external fixator with reduction and internal fixation of the tibia through an as minimally invasive method as possible. A CT scan is used to identify the number of significant fragments and for planning the placement of the incision along a major fracture plane. Also, the direction of internal fixation can be guided by the fracture configuration. This can be done percutaneously or more commonly through a small incision along the ankle joint and the tibial metaphysis.[17,18] An extraperiosteal tunnel is created along the tibia going in a superior direction. An appropriate plate is then applied. There are different plate designs available that are precontoured, malleable, and anatomic specific. The distal screws can be delivered through the plate percutaneously or directly through the incision, whereas the proximal screws can be placed percutaneously. The arthroscope can be used through traditional portals or through the open incision to aid in the reduction of the anterior tibial articular surface and evaluation for osteochondral damage.

Although not commonly done, talar fractures can sometimes be repaired with arthroscopic and fluoroscopic control along with percutaneous screw fixation. This can be done in a fracture that is nondisplaced or very minimally displaced. It is difficult to manipulate the fracture because the talus is compressed between the navicular and the ankle joint.

Last, acute transchondral fractures of the talus may be excised arthroscopically if stage III or IV (see **Fig. 4**B, D, E). The lateral lesion has been described as shallow, wafer-shaped, and located on the more anterior portion of the talar dome. The medial lesion is described as deeper, cup-shaped, and located on the more posterior aspect of the talar dome.[20] Obviously, the lateral talar dome fracture is easier to approach, as it is located more anteriorly. It is also the one more commonly associated with an acute inversion injury of the ankle. Following excision, the talar defect is microfractured. However, significant edema, hemarthrosis, the inability to hold the distending fluid within the ankle capsule, and the rupture of the fibular collateral ligaments may limit

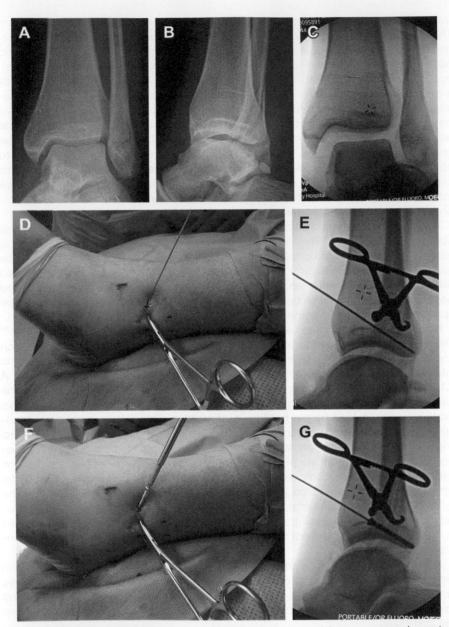

Fig. 6. (A) Mortise and (B) lateral views of Weber B fracture. (C) Stress external rotation x-rays demonstrating lateral talar subluxation. (D, E) Percutaneous reduction of the fibula after initially examining the ankle arthroscopically and finding no articular damage. (F, G) Percutaneous cortical lag screw fixation. (H, I) Percutaneous placement of one-third tubular plate. (J) Percutaneous drilling for screw delivery. (K) AP and (L) lateral views of final ORIF. Fracture reduction is anatomic with good position of the internal fixation. Transyndesmotic screw stabilization of the mortise was necessary.

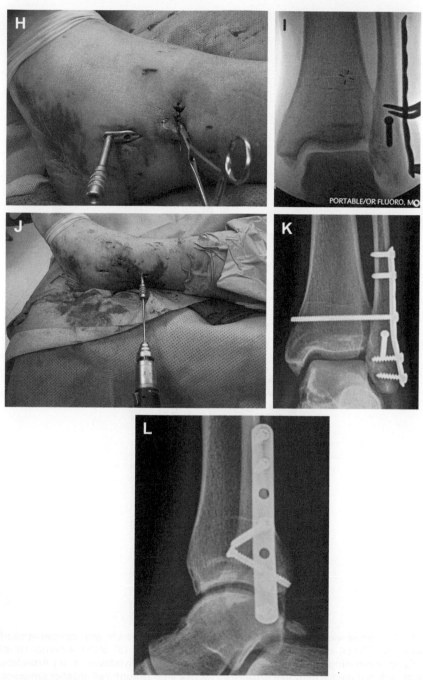

Fig. 6. (*continued*)

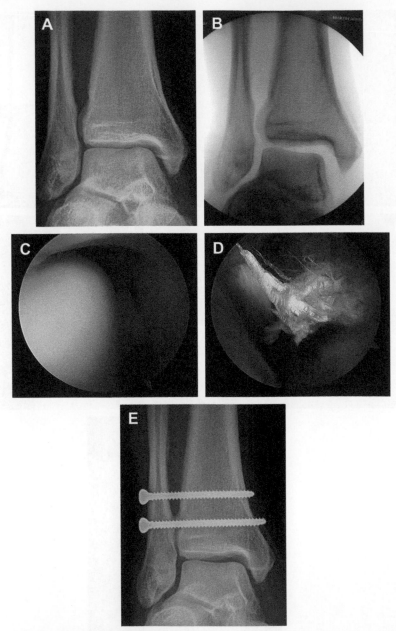

Fig. 7. (*A*) Mortise view of patient who sustained injury to ankle with normal-appearing radiograph. Clinical evaluation indicated possible diastasis. (*B*) Stress external rotation testing demonstrating lateral talar subluxation and widened syndesmosis. (*C*) Arthroscopic view of widened medial joint space. (*D*) Arthroscopic view of ruptured anterior syndesmotic ligament. (*E*) Mortise view demonstrating anatomic reduction of ankle with 2 transdesmotic screws.

this technique. Arthroscopy is more commonly used in the chronic osteochondral lesion.

SUMMARY

Ankle arthroscopy is a valuable tool in the treatment of certain intra-articular fractures involving the ankle, as it provides the ability to address osteochondral injury and aids in the direct visualization for joint reduction through minimal intervention. It can sometimes be complimented by a more minimally invasive approach to fracture reduction and internal fixation. Good indications for a more minimally invasive approach as well as being more flexible in fixation strategies are patients with minimally displaced fractures, specific pediatric fractures, some degree of vascular insufficiency, diabetes, tenuous but not compromised soft tissue situation, or when the anesthesia time needs to be shortened. It should be noted that to perform arthroscopically assisted minimally invasive fracture approaches, the surgeon must have significant experience with traditional open techniques.

REFERENCES

1. Mast JW, Teipner WA. A reproducible approach to the internal fixation of adult ankle fractures: rationale, technique, and early results. Orthop Clin North Am 1980;11:661.
2. Michelson JD. Current concepts review fractures of the ankle. J Bone Joint Surg Am 1990;77:142–52.
3. Ferkel RD, Orwin JF. Ankle arthroscopy: a new tool for treating acute and chronic ankle fractures. Arthroscopy 1993;9:456.
4. Leontaritis N, Hinojosa L, Lauren B, et al. Arthroscopically detected intra-articular lesion associated with acute ankle fractures. J Bone Joint Surg Am 2009;91(2): 333–9.
5. Jupiter JB, Levine AM, Tafton P. Skeletal trauma: basic science, management, and reconstruction. Philadelphia: Elsevier; 2002.
6. Takao M, Ochi M, Shu N, et al. Bandage distraction technique for ankle arthroscopy. Foot Ankle Int 1999;20:389.
7. Spiegel PG, Cooperman DR, Laros GS. Epiphyseal fractures of the distal ends of the tibia and fibula. A retrospective study of 237 cases in children. J Bone Joint Surg Am 1978;60:1046.
8. Kleiger B, Mankin HJ. Fractures of the lateral portion of the distal tibial epiphysis. J Bone Joint Surg Am 1964;46:25.
9. Von Laer L. Classification, diagnosis, and treatment of the transitional fractures of the distal part of the tibia. J Bone Joint Surg Am 1985;67:687.
10. Ert JP, Barrack RL, Alexander AH, et al. Triplane fracture of the distal tibial epiphysis. Long-term follow-up. J Bone Joint Surg Am 1988;70:967.
11. Cooperman DR, Spiegel PG, Laros GS. Tibial Fractures involving the ankle in children: the so-called triplane epiphyseal fracture. J Bone Joint Surg Am 1978; 60:1040.
12. Rapariz JM, Ocete G, Gonzalez-Herranz P, et al. Distal tibial triplane fracture: long-term follow-up. J Pediatr Orthop 1996;16:113.
13. Harper MC. The deltoid ligament: an evaluation of the need for surgical repair. Clin Orthop 1988;226:156.
14. Pankovich AM. Maisonneuve fracture of the fibula. J Bone Joint Surg Am 1976; 58:337.

15. Kaye RA. Stabilization of ankle syndesmosis injuries with a transyndesmotic screw. Foot Ankle 1989;9:290.
16. Sirkin M, Sanders R, DiPasquale T, et al. A staged protocol for soft tissue management in the treatment of complex pilon fractures. J Orthop Trauma 1999;13:78.
17. Patterson MJ, Cole JD. Two-staged delayed open reduction and internal fixation of severe pilon fractures. J Orthop Trauma 1999;13:85.
18. Helfet DL, Shonnard PY, Levine D, et al. Minimally invasive plate osteosynthesis of distal tibial fractures. Injury 1997;28(Suppl 1):42.
19. Salton HL, Rush S, Schuberth J. Tibial plafond fractures: limited incision reduction with percutaneous fixation. J Foot Ankle Surg 2007;46(4):261.
20. Berndt A, Harty M. Transchondral fractures (osteochondritis dissecans) of the talus. J Bone Joint Surg Am 1959;41:988.

Subtalar Joint Arthroscopy

Laurence G. Rubin, DPM

KEYWORDS

• Subtalar • Arthroscopy • Portals

Although the subtalar and ankle joints are related by proximity, they are different anatomically. The anatomy of the subtalar joint presents challenges even to an experienced arthroscopist. The subtalar joint has 4 joint surfaces, and they are all not contiguous: the posterior facet, middle facet, anterior facet, and the talonavicular joint. There are intra-articular and periarticular ligaments. The roots of the extensor retinaculum are also intra-articular and must be navigated around during a subtalar arthroscopy.

The posterior portion of the subtalar joint can also be entered, and surgery can be performed in this region. This area presents its own unique set of challenges. The capsule is more tightly approximated to the articular surfaces. The distal aspect of the talus comes to a narrow end, leaving only several millimeters between the articular surfaces of the subtalar and ankle joints. Diagnostic and therapeutic indications for subtalar joint arthroscopy have increased in the recent past. This article covers the basic technique of subtalar joint arthroscopy and some of the more advanced indications.

DIAGNOSTIC TESTS

Correct diagnosis of an intra-articular pathologic process is one of the most important aspects of a successful subtalar joint arthroscopy. The first step is a thorough clinical examination for making sure that pathology in the following structures has been ruled out: ankle joint, lateral gutter of the ankle, peroneal tendons, calcaneal-cuboid joint, lateral ankle ligaments, and the sural nerve. Radiographs are often of limited value. They can be helpful in diagnosing arthritic conditions and coalitions, but radiographic findings for these conditions become evident later in the disease process.

One of the most beneficial diagnostic tests is a selective block of the subtalar joint. The patient is prepared and injected into the sinus tarsi/subtalar joint with ropivacaine. Marcaine can also be used, but there is concern for chondrocyte toxicity.[1] The patient is instructed to resume normal activities with attention to those activities that they could not perform before the block. An intracapsular problem should achieve significant-to-total relief of symptoms from the block.

Private Practice, 3808 Hackamore Lane, Richmond, VA 23233, USA
E-mail address: lgrubin@comcast.net

Clin Podiatr Med Surg 28 (2011) 539–550
doi:10.1016/j.cpm.2011.05.005
0891-8422/11/$ – see front matter © 2011 Elsevier Inc. All rights reserved.

Diagnostic tests such as computed tomographic scans, bone scans, and magnetic resonance imaging (MRI) can be used but may have limited diagnostic value. Goldberger and Conti[2] concluded that arthroscopy of the subtalar joint was "the most accurate method of diagnosing subtalar articular cartilage damage ..." Their study compared plain radiographs, MRI, bone scans, and intraoperative findings of subtalar joint arthroscopy. Lee and colleagues[3] concluded that MRI was effective for determining cervical ligament tears, alterations of fat within the sinus tarsi, and synovial thickening but was inaccurate in correctly detecting interosseous ligament tears. Oloff and colleagues[4] reported that "magnetic resonance imaging was useful in identifying subtalar joint chronic synovitis and/or fibrosis in all 26 patients who were imaged."

CONSERVATIVE TREATMENT

Subtalar joint pathology is usually a late finding on presentation to the surgeon. There is frequently an inflammatory component of the process at the initial presentation, and therefore, immobilization of the joint is usually best performed in combination with an attempt to decrease the intra-articular inflammatory process. A nonsteroidal antiinflammatory drug or an oral steroid is frequently prescribed at the initial visit. Subsequent conservative treatments can include intra-articular injections with an anesthetic and cortisone. Physical therapy can also be used. Joint mobilization and phonophoresis are often helpful in the treatment of subtalar joint pathology.

RESULTS

Subtalar joint arthroscopy has high patient satisfaction rates, with minimal complications. Williams and Ferkel[5] reported 86% good-to-excellent results in a subgroup of 29 patients, all with demonstrable arthroscopic pathology. Ahn and colleagues[6] reported on 115 consecutive patients who underwent arthroscopy. This study was performed on a wide variety of cases, including arthroscopic subtalar arthrodesis, and found a 97% patient satisfaction rate, with no serious complications reported. Frey and colleagues[7] reviewed 49 subtalar arthroscopies, with an average follow-up of more than 4 years. Their excellent-to-good results were 94%, with all the patients with 6% poor result eventually having successful subtalar joint arthrodesis. There were 5 reported complications of the 49 procedures. There were no reported complications in the study by Williams and Ferkel[5] or Goldberger and Conti.[2]

INSTRUMENTATION

The diameter of the arthroscope, for the subtalar joint, varies from 1.9, 2.7, to 4.0 mm. The surgeon can also choose between a 30° and a 70° lens. Synovial resectors are frequently used to debride tissue and range in diameter from 2.7 to 4.0 mm. Thermal ablation is another commonly used modality. It allows debridement and arthroscopic coagulation. The newer products have suction built into the tip that prevents a buildup of intra-articular bubbles and safeguards to prevent overheating of the fluid inside the joint.

Subtalar joint arthroscopy can be performed with or without distraction. Invasive distraction is rarely used but can be achieved with the use of a monolateral external fixator. The distal arm of the fixator is rotated allowing both pins to enter the calcaneus. Noninvasive distraction can be accomplished by tying Kerlix around the patient's subtalar joint and around the surgeon's waist. The surgeon leans back, creating distraction at the joint. There are also several commercial noninvasive distractors on the market. Noninvasive distraction is a 3-part system. It consists of a leg holder, the distraction apparatus that attaches to the operating table, and a heel strap. Because of the nature of the procedure, the skin is wet and the strap from the noninvasive distractor can frequently slip off the back of the heel. Mastisol, placed on the heel, will help prevent the strap from slipping, but if this continues, minimally invasive distraction will prevent the heel strap from slipping. A 0.62 inches Kirschner wire is placed transversely across the calcaneus, and the posterior strap is placed over the wire (**Figs. 1** and **2**). Wires larger than 0.62 inches can create too much traction. This has produced neuritis specifically at the deep and superficial peroneal nerves.

PROCEDURE

The patient is placed on the operating table in the supine position. This can also be done in the lateral decubitus position. For posterior subtalar joint arthroscopy, the patient is placed in a lateral decubitus or prone position. The tower or viewing platform is placed on the contralateral side of the patient for the supine approach.

The portals are marked before insufflation to prevent losing the anatomic boundaries once the joint is distended (**Fig. 3**). The subtalar joint can be approached through several portals: lateral, accessory lateral, medial,[8] middle,[9] posteromedial, and posterolateral.[10] The author's preferred technique is to use anterolateral and middle portals. These portals are easily developed by palpating into the sinus tarsi, anterior to the fibula, and posterior to the beak of the calcaneus (**Figs. 4–6**). When a posterior approach is needed, a switch stick is used in the middle portal. This technique is visualized through the anterolateral portal. Once the position of the portal has been determined by the switch stick's protrusion on the posterolateral aspect of the ankle/subtalar joint, a small incision is made over the protruding switch stick and an arthroscopic cannula is then placed over the switch stick (**Figs. 7** and **8**). This allows direct access to the posterior aspect of the subtalar joint. A 70° arthroscope is placed into the middle portal for visualization, whereas the posterolateral portal is used as a working portal.

One of the complications of portal placement is damage to the surrounding structures. Tryfonidis and colleagues[11] compared the distance from the sural nerve to the traditional portals for subtalar joint arthroscopy: anterior, middle, and posterior. The study concluded that the distances from the anterior, middle, and posterior portals to the nearest nerve were 21.3, 20.9, and 11.4 mm, respectively. Frey and colleagues[9] evaluated the distance from the portals to the surrounding structures.

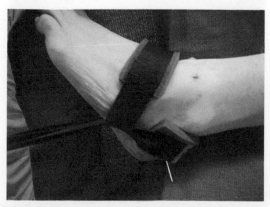

Fig. 1. Semi-invasive ankle distraction with a 0.62 inches Kirschner wire.

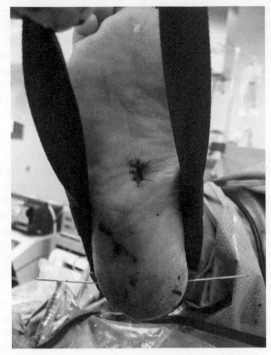

Fig. 2. Semi-invasive ankle distraction with a 0.62 inches Kirschner wire.

The anterior portal was at an average distance of 17 mm from the dorsal intermediate cutaneous branch, 8 mm from a branch off the sural nerve, 21 mm from the peroneus tertius tendon but only 2 mm from a branch off the lesser saphenous vein. The posterior portal was at an average distance of 4 mm from the sural nerve, 11 mm from the

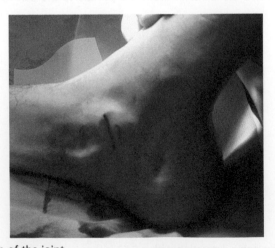

Fig. 3. Insufflation of the joint.

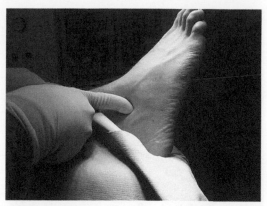

Fig. 4. Palpating the sinus tarsi.

peroneal tendons, and 15 mm from the Achilles tendon. Once the subtalar joint is entered, the surgeon can perform an inspection of the intra-articular structures (**Figs. 9–12**). Debridement of the joint is performed using synovial resectors, thermal ablation, suction punches, and curettes.

PATHOLOGY

Sinus tarsi syndrome is the most distinctive diagnosis of the subtalar joint. Oloff and colleagues[4] found subtalar joint arthroscopy to be safe and effective in the diagnosis and treatment of sinus tarsi syndrome. In their study of 29 patients, 12 patients required 15 additional surgeries. Frey and colleagues[7] reported on a subgroup of 14 feet with a preoperative diagnosis of sinus tarsi syndrome. At the time of arthroscopy, all 14 diagnoses were revised. Ten patients were diagnosed with interosseous ligament tears, 2 with arthrofibrosis, and 2 with joint degeneration. They concluded that sinus tarsi syndrome was not an accurate term, and a more specific diagnosis should be made. Lee and colleagues[12] evaluated 33 consecutive procedures on 31 patients with sinus tarsi syndrome. Postoperative findings showed a partial tear of the

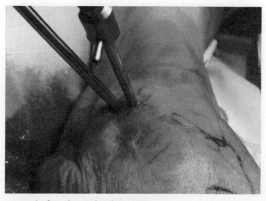

Fig. 5. Arthroscopic portals for the subtalar joint.

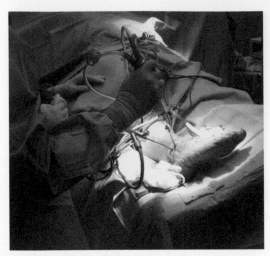

Fig. 6. Arthroscopic portals for the subtalar joint.

interosseous ligament in 29, synovitis in 18, partial tear of the cervical ligament in 11, arthrofibrosis in 8, and soft tissue impingement in 7 patients. They concluded that arthroscopy identified intra-articular pathology in patients with sinus tarsi syndrome. Patients in this study reported 40% excellent results, 39% good results, and 12% fair results.

Field and Ng[13] described the resection of the middle facet using subtalar joint arthroscopy. The os trigonum can also be resected arthroscopically, which can be performed with the patient in a lateral decubitus position. A 70° scope is placed in the lateral portal, and the posterolateral portal is the instrument portal. This can also be achieved with the patient in a prone position through posteromedial and posterolateral portals or with a posterolateral and an accessory posterolateral portal.[14] Horibe and colleagues[14] had excellent results and no complications in 11 patients of arthroscopic os trigonum excision.

One of the most common diagnoses encountered in subtalar joint arthroscopy is tearing and impingement of the interosseous ligament. This diagnosis can be

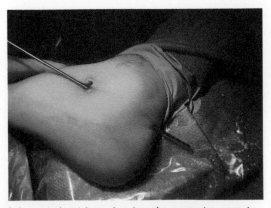

Fig. 7. Placement of the switch stick to develop the posterior portal.

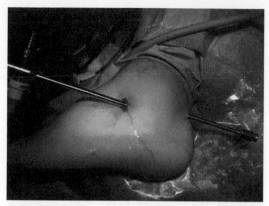

Fig. 8. Inserting the cannula over the switch stick.

challenging, because there is no objective diagnostic testing that will allow for an accurate diagnosis. As previously stated in Lee's study,[3] MRI is inaccurate for diagnosing interosseous ligament tears. Frey and colleagues[7] found that 36 of 49 arthroscopies were diagnosed with an intraosseous ligament tear and that 27 of those patients had impingement into the anterior aspect of the posterior articulation. Lee and colleagues[12] diagnosed 88% of 33 patients with sinus tarsi syndrome with an impingement lesion postoperatively. Impingement lesions are commonly found in the anteromedial portion of the posterior articulation of the subtalar joint. A distinct tear of the interosseous ligament may or may not be present. The lesion can be debrided using a synovial resector or suction punch (**Fig. 13**). Care should be taken to avoid damage to the interosseous ligament and the posterior and medial articular facets during debridement.

Another area that soft tissue debridement has been useful is the removal of arthroereisis implants. The implant is identified inside the sinus tarsi. A careful removal is performed rather than a blind disruption of the soft tissues. The resulting synovitis and fibrosis that were caused by the arthroereisis are debrided at the same time

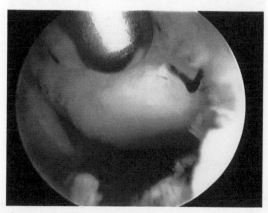

Fig. 9. The anterior facet and plantar lateral aspect of the talonavicular joint.

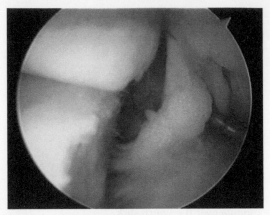

Fig. 10. The lateral aspect of the posterior facet.

(**Fig. 14**). This has proven to be particularly beneficial in adults requiring an arthroereisis explantation.

Several authors describe debridement of the subtalar joint after intra-articular calcaneal fractures. Elgafy and Ebraheim[15] reported on 10 consecutive patients. Eight patients had significant pain relief and did not require further injection therapy or surgery, whereas 2 required an arthrodesis. Lee and colleagues[16] followed up 17 patients with a mean follow-up of 16.8 months after arthroscopic release for subtalar joint stiffness from the intra-articular fractures. All patients reported increased movement of the subtalar joint with no complications. Of the 17 patients, 6 were very satisfied, 8 were satisfied, and 3 were not satisfied with their outcome. Two of their patients required a fusion. This procedure is technically challenging because of the intracapsular fibrosis and requires extensive debridement of the soft tissues between and around the articular surfaces (**Fig. 15**). The fibrosis can create a white out and prevent the surgeon from being able to see any normal anatomy at the onset of the procedure. It can also prevent the ability to distract the joint.

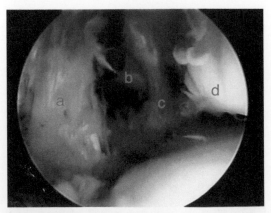

Fig. 11. (a) Cervical ligament, (b) middle facet, (c) interosseous ligament, and (d) posterior facet.

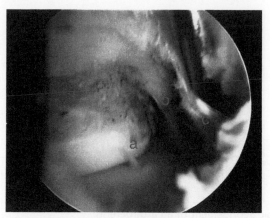

Fig. 12. (a) Posterior facet, (b) interosseous ligament, and (c) retinaculum.

Arthroscopy of the subtalar joint to assist in the reduction and percutaneous fixation of intra-articular calcaneal fractures has also been described in the literature. In 2002, Gavlik and colleagues[17] found that arthroscopy was able to detect incongruencies of the posterior facet in more than 25% of 47 intra-articular calcaneal fractures that appeared to be correctly reduced intraoperatively by fluoroscopy. The same authors[18] reported that 22% of 59 intra-articular fractures were found to have a 1- to 2-mm

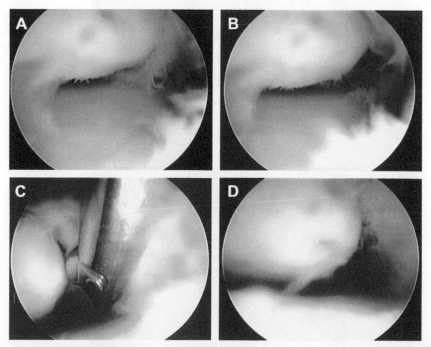

Fig. 13. (A) Impingement lesion. (B) Synovitis at the impingement. (C) Debridement with a suction punch. (D) Complete debridement of the lesion.

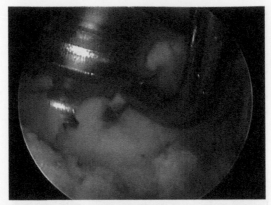

Fig. 14. Arthroscopic debridement of an arthroereisis.

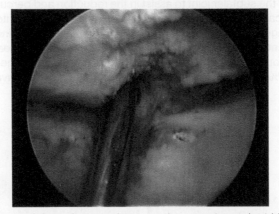

Fig. 15. Debridement of the soft tissues between the posterior and middle facets.

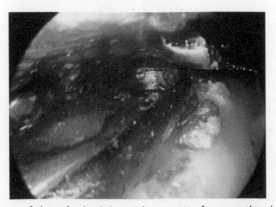

Fig. 16. Debridement of the subtalar joint with a curette for an arthrodesis.

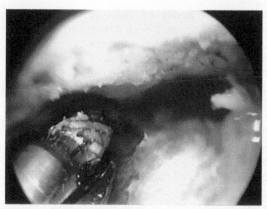

Fig. 17. Debridement of the subtalar joint with a burr for an arthrodesis.

step-off detected after visual and fluoroscopic evaluations of the reduction. Eighteen patients in that study with a Sanders II had arthroscopically assisted percutaneous reduction and screw fixation; 15 of those were reevaluated after 1 year with excellent clinical results. Schuberth and colleagues[19] reported on minimally invasive arthroscopic-assisted reduction and fixation in 24 patients. They reported no soft tissue complications, and of the 18 patients who were followed up for more than 1 year, none had a subtalar joint fusion.

Subtalar joint arthrodesis can be performed arthroscopically. This has been described from an anterior and a posterior approach. The contraindications are significant deformity and bone loss. The procedure has high rates of fusion with minimal complications and can be performed with or without distraction. Curettes and arthroscopic burrs are used to debride the cartilage and subchondral bone (**Figs. 16** and **17**). Fixation of the fusion is the same as the open procedure. Glanzmann and Sanhueza-Hernandez[20] reported a 100% fusion rate on 41 procedures performed on 37 consecutive patients. Amendola and colleagues[21] fused 11 joints in 10 patients and reported 1 nonunion, with 8 of the 10 patients being very satisfied with their surgery.

SUMMARY

Subtalar joint arthroscopy can be performed on a wide array of pathology. The procedure has progressed from a diagnostic test to a reconstructive procedure. Although it is not as popular as ankle arthroscopy, it is becoming more commonly discussed in the literature and is part of many arthroscopy courses. Better education along with improved instrumentation will allow more foot and ankle surgeons to treat pathology of the subtalar joint with arthroscopic techniques. This will lead to improved outcomes and lower complication rates in treating that pathology.

REFERENCES

1. Piper SL, Kim HT. Comparison of ropivacaine and bupivacaine toxicity in human articular chondrocytes. J Bone Joint Surg Am 2008;90(5):986–91.
2. Goldberger MI, Conti SF. Clinical outcome after subtalar arthroscopy. Foot Ankle Int 1998;19(7):462–5.
3. Lee KB, Bai LB, Park JG, et al. Efficacy of MRI versus arthroscopy for evaluation of sinus tarsi syndrome. Foot Ankle Int 2008;29(11):1111–6.

4. Oloff LM, Schulhofer SD, Bocko AP. Subtalar joint arthroscopy for sinus tarsi syndrome: a review of 29 cases. J Foot Ankle Surg 2001;40(3):152–7.
5. Williams MM, Ferkel RD. Subtalar arthroscopy: indications, technique, and results. Foot Ankle Int 1998;14(4):373–81.
6. Ahn JH, Lee JH, Kim KJ, et al. Subtalar arthroscopic procedures for the treatment of subtalar pathologic conditions: 115 consecutive cases. Orthopedics 2009; 32(12):891–6.
7. Frey C, Feder KS, DiGiovanni C. Arthroscopic evaluation of the subtalar joint: the sinus tarsi syndrome exist? Foot Ankle Int 1999;20:185–91.
8. Mekhail AO, Heck BE, Ebraheim NA, et al. Arthroscopy of the subtalar joint: establishing a medial portal. Foot Ankle Int 1995;16:427–32.
9. Frey C, Gasser S, Feder K. Arthroscopy of the subtalar joint. Foot Ankle Int 1994; 15:424–8.
10. Phisitkul P, Tochigi Y, Saltzman CL, et al. Arthroscopic visualization of the posterior subtalar joint in the prone position: cadaver study. Arthroscopy 2006;22(5): 511–5.
11. Tryfonidis M, Whitefield CG, Charalambous CP, et al. The distance between the sural nerve and ideal portal placements and lateral subtalar arthroscopy: a cadaveric study. Foot Ankle Int 2008;29(8):842–4.
12. Lee KB, Bai LB, Song EK, et al. Subtalar arthroscopy for sinus tarsi syndrome: arthroscopic findings and clinical outcomes of 33 consecutive cases. Arthroscopy 2008;24(10):1130–4.
13. Field C, Ng A. Resection of middle facet collection is arthroscopic guidance. J Foot Ankle Surg 2009;48(2):273–6.
14. Horibe S, Kita K, Natsu-ume T, et al. A novel technique of arthroscopic excision of a symptomatic os trigonum. Arthroscopy 2008;24(1):121.e1–4.
15. Elgafy H, Ebraheim NA. Subtalar arthroscopy for persistent sub-fibular pain after calcaneal fractures. Foot Ankle Int 1999;20(7):422–7.
16. Lee KB, Chung JY, Song EK, et al. Arthroscopic release for painful subtalar stiffness after intra-articular fractures of the calcaneum. J Bone Joint Surg Br 2008; 90(11):1457–61.
17. Gavlik JM, Rammelt S, Zwipp H. The use of subtalar arthroscopy in open reduction and internal fixation of intra-articular calcaneal fractures. Injury 2002;33(1): 63–71.
18. Rammelt S, Gavlik JM, Barthel S, et al. The value of subtalar arthroscopy in the management of intra-articular calcaneal fractures. Foot Ankle Int 2002;23(10): 906–16.
19. Schuberth JM, Cobb MD, Talarico RH. Minimally invasive arthroscopic-assisted reduction with percutaneous fixation in the management of intra-articular calcaneal fractures: a review of 24 cases. J Foot Ankle Surg 2009;48(3):315–22.
20. Glanzmann MC, Sanhueza-Hernandez R. Arthroscopic subtalar arthrodesis for symptomatic osteoarthritis of the hindfoot: a prospective study of 41 cases. Foot Ankle Int 2007;28(1):2–7.
21. Amendola A, Lee KB, Saltzman CL, et al. Technique and early experience with posterior arthroscopic subtalar arthrodesis. Foot Ankle Int 2007;28(3):298–302.

Small Joint Arthroscopy of the Foot

Richard Derner, DPM[a],*, Jason Naldo, DPM[b]

KEYWORDS

- Arthroscopy • Small joints • Foot
- First metatarsophalangeal joint

The arthroscopic approach to small joints of the foot has made many advances in recent years, which can be directly related to the improvement of the surgical equipment. This improvement has led to more indications for the use of arthroscopy as well as minimizing the complications. Several articles recently have presented experiences arthroscopic surgery in the small joints of the foot; however, its use is still relatively limited. Approaches to small joints of the foot involve the first metatarsophalangeal, tarsometatarsal, and the Chopart joint, as well as the interphalangeal joint to the great toe and lesser toes.

HISTORY

Arthroscopic treatment of the first metatarsophalangeal joint was first described by Wanatabe[1] in 1972. Bartlett[2] first reported its use in 1988. In 2006 Debnath and colleagues[3] noted 95% of patients remaining pain-free at 2 years following first metatarsophalangeal joint (MTPJ) arthroscopy for treatment of early signs of degenerative joint disease. In 2008 Lui[4] demonstrated a statistically significant correlation between joint cartilage erosion, joint synovitis, and pain in hallux valgus. He also noted a statistically significant correlation between the size of cartilage defect and severity of hallux valgus using diagnostic arthroscopy of the first MTPJ.[4] In 2009 Wang and colleagues[5] noted a statistically significant decrease in recurrence of acute gouty arthritis to the first MTPJ following arthroscopic debridement of tophi when compared with patients treated by medical means alone. Liu and colleagues[6] has reported on performing arthroscopy on the great toe joint for hallux valgus deformity, with good results. These investigators evaluated 94 feet treated for hallux valgus deformity and felt that arthroscopy can be effective in improving both clinical and radiographic findings in patients with appropriate indications. These findings included a reducible first intermetatarsal angle and no significant deformity to the distal first metatarsal articular angle. Patients were treated with an endoscopic soft tissue release and medial exostectomy; proximal

[a] Private Practice, Associated Foot & Ankle Centers of Northern Virginia, Lake Ridge, VA, USA
[b] Inova Fairfax Hospital, Department of Orthopaedics, Section of Podiatry, Falls Church, VA, USA
* Corresponding author.
E-mail address: richd87@aol.com

Clin Podiatr Med Surg 28 (2011) 551–560
doi:10.1016/j.cpm.2011.05.004
0891-8422/11/$ – see front matter © 2011 Published by Elsevier Inc.

screw placement after manual manipulation was performed to close the intermetatarsal angle. An endoscopic approach to soft tissue release at the first MTPJ for treatment of hallux valgus has also been reported, with a significant increase in American Orthopaedic Foot and Ankle Society (AOFAS) score at greater than 2 years of follow up.[6]

The use of arthroscopic technology for small joints of the foot has not been limited to the diagnosis and treatment of first MTPJ pathology. Arthrodesis of the first metatarsocuneiform (MCJ) joint through a plantar-medial and dorsal-medial portal system has been recently described.[7] In 2007 Lui[8] presented a tarsometatarsal (Lisfranc) joint arthrodesis following a neglected fracture/dislocation through a 5-portal dorsal approach. Parisien and Vangsness[9] first reported the arthroscopic approach to subtalar joint deformity in 1985, but the calcaneocuboid and talonavicular joint resection for triple arthrodesis by arthroscopic means was also demonstrated by Lui[10] in 2006. In 2010 Bauer and colleagues[11] reported the first case of calcaneonavicular coalition resection by endoscopic means, resulting in an AOFAS score of 82 at 2 years of follow up.

ANATOMY

To properly perform arthroscopic procedures to the small joints of the foot, a firm understanding of the anatomy of these joints is required. In describing the first MTPJ complex, the base of the proximal phalanx of the hallux is ovoid in shape; wider than it is tall, concave both medial to lateral as well as dorsal to plantar. Little stability is gained from the chondroid nature of the first MTPJ, due to shallow surface for articulation between the phalanx and the metatarsal head.[12] The rounded head of the first metatarsal has a side-to-side curvature that is greater than the vertical curvature and is somewhat wider (20–24 mm) than its height (16–20 mm).[13] The articular surface, covered by hyaline cartilage, extends onto the dorsal aspect of the metatarsal head and continues plantarly into the medial and lateral grooves, which serve as articulations for the sesamoid bones, with the medial groove larger and deeper to accommodate for the larger tibial sesamoid. The plantar grooves are separated by a median crest, known as the crista.[13] The joint capsule of the first MTPJ attaches close to cartilaginous edges dorsally; however, plantarly it attaches several millimeters proximal to the cartilage, with the plantar aspect of the capsule thicker than the dorsal capsule because of the presence of the plantar metatarsophalangeal ligament. The metatarsosesamoid ligaments thicken the medial and lateral aspects of the joint capsule, along with the medial and lateral collateral ligaments, which tract from the medial and lateral metatarsal tubercles to the corresponding tubercles on the sides of the phalanx (**Fig. 1**).[13] The sesamoid bones of the flexor hallucis brevis muscle, which ossify

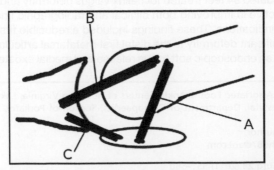

Fig. 1. A, metatarsosesamoidal (suspensory) ligament; B, metatarsophalangeal collateral ligament; C, phalangeal-sesamoidal ligament.

between 10 and 12 years of age, are attached to the metatarsal via the metatarsose-samoidal ligaments and to the proximal phalanx of the hallux via the phalangeal-sesamoidal ligaments, respectively. The sesamoids also firmly adhere to the plantar metatarsophalangeal ligament, which results in a firm attachment to the proximal phalanx. The sesamoids therefore do not move relative to the proximal phalanx but relative to the metatarsal. Along with the ligamentous attachments already described, there are tendon attachments to the sesamoid bones as well. The tibial sesamoid provides an insertion point for the abductor hallucis, and the fibular sesamoid provides an insertion point for the adductor hallucis as well as the deep transverse metatarsal ligament. Contraction of the soft tissues that insert on the fibular sesamoid have been reported to contribute to the formation of hallux abducto valgus.[14]

The first MCJ is the largest of the tarsometatarsal joints. The outline of the facets of the first MCJ is reniform in shape with the hilus laterally. The articular surface of the base of the first metatarsal is 25 to 30 mm deep and 16 to 20 mm wide, and the surface is concave dorsally and flat or slightly convex in the more plantar aspect of the joint.[15] The corresponding dorsal part of the distal aspect of the medial cuneiform is slightly convex, with the plantar aspect flat or slightly concave, allowing for inversion and eversion along the long axis of the metatarsal.

The midtarsal joint comprises the talonavicular joint (TNJ) and the calcaneocuboid joint (CCJ). The TNJ is condylar in nature while the CCJ is a saddle joint. These joints cannot act independently, as motion in the subtalar joint (STJ) and CCJ is required for motion at the TNJ. The head of the talus is convex in all directions and bears at least 3 recognizable articular areas: an ovoid area for articulation with the navicular, a trian-gular facet for the plantar calcaneonavicular ligament, and a long oval area plantarly for the anterior calcaneal articular facet. The posterior surface of the navicular is ovoid in shape, broader laterally than medially; the articular surface is concave and wholly articular with the head of the talus. The talonavicular ligament is a wide, thin band that connects the superior surface of the talar neck to the dorsal surface of the navic-ular. The calcaneonavicular ligament component of the bifurcate ligament also serves to provide medial support to the calcaneocuboid joint and lateral support to the TNJ. The anterior surface of the calcaneus is shaped roughly like an inverted triangle. The articular surface is concave from superior to inferior and convex transversely, giving the characteristic saddle shape. The posterior surface of the cuboid has a saddle shape corresponding to the anterior surface of the calcaneus.[13]

PHYSICAL EXAMINATION

Physical examination of the first MTPJ should include open and closed chain range of motion, and inspection for a soft or hard end point of range of motion. Examination for crepitus should be done and pain along the joint line should be noted. Dorsiflexion range of motion should be greater than 60° in both the open and closed chain. If a hard end point of dorsiflexion is noted with decreased range of motion, dorsal osteo-phyte formation is most likely the cause. On forced dorsiflexion, pain is usually elicited as a result of bony impingement between the dorsal metatarsal and proximal phalanx osteophytes. If pain is a result of forced plantarflexion, stretching of the extensor hal-lucis longus tendon, MTPJ capsule, and inflamed synovium are usually the instigating factors.[16] Crepitus, or the feeling of grinding or clicking in the joint on motion, is typical with extensive cartilage erosion. If decreased range of motion in the first MTPJ is noted, hypermobility at the first MCJ must be inspected. Hypermobility can be tested by stabilizing the lateral forefoot in one hand, while gripping the first metatarsal neck in other and assessing sagittal and transverse plane motion.[12] Lastly, examination of the sesamoids with direct palpation and through range of motion is important in determining the cause of pain before proceeding with surgery.

DIAGNOSTIC MODALITIES

Various radiographic studies can be used to aid in diagnosis and decision making for operative treatment. Weight-bearing anteroposterior (AP) and lateral radiographs can be very useful in diagnosing early-onset hallux rigidus (**Fig. 2**). The presence of joint space narrowing, medial and lateral osteophyte formation, and sesamoid hypertrophy on the AP radiograph aid in assessing the extent of disease in the joint. The extent of dorsal osteophyte formation noted on lateral radiograph can assist the surgeon when deciding whether an arthroscopic or open treatment is indicated. In the absence of plain film radiographic findings in the symptomatic patient, further studies can be performed to aid in diagnosis and treatment. The use of computed tomography scans and magnetic resonance imaging can provide information about osteochondral defects or other underlying pathology (**Fig. 3**).[16]

INDICATIONS FOR ARTHROSCOPIC TREATMENT

Arthroscopy of the first MTPJ has become more common, but its use is still limited in comparison with other joints in the body. Specific indications for arthroscopy of this joint include osteochondral lesions, synovitis, early degenerative changes, loose bodies, and arthrofibrosis. Osteophytes limiting dorsiflexion of the great toe joint can be treated arthroscopically and are usually smaller than 5 mm. Anything larger than 5 mm is typically treated with open resection via cheilectomy. Less common use of first MTPJ arthroscopy is evaluation and treatment of sesamoid pathology; excision of gouty tophi can also be performed for this joint. Overall, indications for

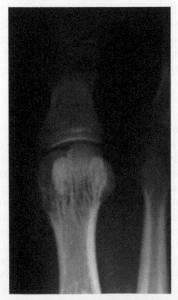

Fig. 2. Plain film radiograph. Dorsoplantar view of an osteochondral defect within the first metatarsal head.

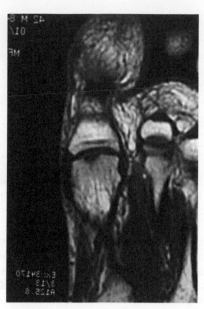

Fig. 3. Magnetic resonance image confirming the osteochondral lesion to the first metatarsal head.

performing arthroscopy of the great toe joint are based on clinical symptoms as well as radiographic findings.

Contraindications include severe joint arthrosis, arterial insufficiency, and other specific joint pathology, which can be better treated with the open technique.

PREOPERATIVE PLANNING

Before performing a first MTPJ arthroscopy, several things must be considered for a successful surgical outcome. Due to the size of this joint, appropriate equipment is mandatory for both visualization and treatment of the joint arthroscopically. The first MTPJ is typically visualized with either a 1.9-mm or 2.3-mm arthroscope, which allows for good visualization and enough room for the treatment of the pathology within this joint. A small shaver and abrader also are used for most arthroscopic procedures. Distraction of this joint can be done in one of two ways. Manual distraction by the assistant when necessary is sometimes all that is needed to inspect and treat the great toe joint. However, in more challenging situations a mini external fixator can be employed to help with distraction of this joint (**Fig. 4**).

FIRST MTPJ ARTHROSCOPIC TECHNIQUE

The patient is placed in the supine position on the operating table and the anesthesia department administers intravenous sedation. A sterile pneumatic ankle tourniquet is typically used and applied above the ankle. The great toe is distracted, and a puckering at the joint confirms placement of the portals both dorsomedially and dorsolaterally (**Fig. 5**). A small incision is made longitudinally medial to the extensor hallucis longus (EHL) tendon. Blunt dissection is carried down to the joint to avoid neurovascular injury, and the joint is then insufflated with approximately 5 mL of lactated Ringer solution (**Fig. 6**). As the toe is distracted, a blunt obturator is placed into the dorsomedial

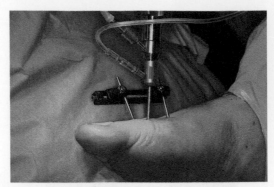

Fig. 4. The use of a mini external fixator to distract the first MTPJ to aid in visualization within the great toe joint.

portal and then into the joint, followed by the arthroscope. Most commonly, a 2.3-mm arthroscope with a 30° angulation is used for the first MTPJ, which gives good visualization into the joint and allows for ease of movement within the joint. A second incision is then made lateral to the EHL tendon and a needle is used initially for outflow. A mid-medial incision may be employed to gain access to the plantar portion of the joint. This action can aid in removing debris plantarly and evaluating lesions to the joint.

A blunt obturator is then used to enter the dorsolateral portal to allow for better egress of fluid and placement of instruments. The joint is then inspected and a 2-mm probe is employed to evaluate the cartilage surface, look for lesions, and inspect the synovial recesses. A 1.9- to 2.0-mm shaver or thermocoagulator may be required to remove both hypertrophic and hemorrhagic synovitis within the joint, including the medial and plantar synovial proliferations. This action permits better visualization within the joint.

Inspection of the joint proceeds in a clockwise pattern starting at the dorsal central aspect of the metatarsal head, then laterally to the superior lateral surface, into the lateral gutter, the central aspect of the first metatarsal head, then medially to the gutter and inferiorly to the tibial sesamoid-metatarsal joint. The proximal phalanx is then evaluated as well. The distal recesses medially, and articular surface of the base of the proximal phalanx laterally, are then evaluated as well. Traction is applied to the great toe either by an assistant or if necessary by a mini external fixator. Although invasive,

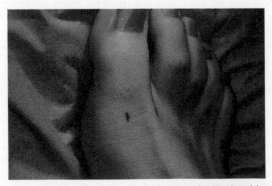

Fig. 5. The dorsomedial and dorsolateral portal sites are determined by distracting the toe and visualizing the puckering within the great toe joint. Care must be taken to avoid the neurovascular structures with portal placement.

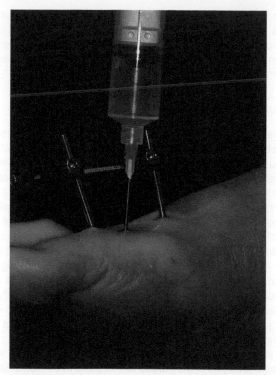

Fig. 6. Use of lactated Ringer solution to insufflate the joint prior to entrance into the joint with the blunt obturator.

this latter technique gives excellent distraction of the great toe joint. If necessary an articulating external fixator arm can give plantarflexion at the same time as distraction, to allow easier evaluation of the plantar structures. The arthroscope is then placed into the dorsolateral portal to visualize the plantar fibular sesamoid-metatarsal joint. At this point, any obvious lesions are identified and removed via curettes, creating sharp borders of cartilage. A 0.035-inch Kirschner wire is then used to microfracture the subchondral bone plate. Meniscoid bodies that are identified are then removed with a small basket and cutters as necessary. Fibrous bands are also excised using a similar technique. Care should be taken plantarly to avoid injuring the sesamoid articulation and joint.

Small joint cutting blades and graspers as well as a thermocoagulator can be used in this second portal.

ADVANTAGES

There are several advantages to first MTPJ arthroscopy; these include all that are common with any other arthroscopic procedure. Minimizing soft tissue dissection, decreased postoperative pain, small capsular incisions, decreased stiffness, and early return to function are all benefits of first MTPJ arthroscopy.

COMPLICATIONS

Complications related to first MTPJ arthroscopy is uncommon, and one needs to be a skilled arthroscopic surgeon to minimize their occurrence. Poor portal placement can lead to nerve injury, either transection or neuropraxia. Cutting of the EHL tendon can also occur as a result of poor handling of the sharp trocars and instruments. Soft tissue swelling and long-term joint effusion can also occur in these patients. Persistent pain, stiffness, and complex regional pain syndrome can occur, as with any other surgery performed on the foot and ankle.

TARSOMETATARSAL JOINT ARTHROSCOPY

Very little has been written on the arthroscopy of the tarsometatarsal joint. Lui[8] has described the fusion of the first MCJ after Lisfranc fracture dislocation. Five portals were used to visualize these joints. Medially for the first MCJ, between the first and second metatarsals and medial cuneiform; the second MCJ is accessed via a portal at the junction of the central cuneiform bone and second and third metatarsals; the third and fourth metatarsal-tarsal joints are visualized via a portal between these bones and the lateral cuneiform and cuboid bone; and the fifth portal is at the junction of the cuboid and fourth and fifth metatarsal bases. Liu also noted that because fusion of the lateral column is rarely performed, tendon arthroplasty could be undertaken.

To date there has been little written in the literature regarding this technique. However, minimizing dissection and preserving vascular supply has a definite benefit for any arthroscopic arthrodesis. This advantage has been frequently identified when fusing the ankle arthroscopically.[17,18] One has to be very skilled to identify and gain access to these joints arthroscopically because there is usually a large degree of osteophytic lipping and joint space narrowing.

Arthroscopic fusion alone of the first MCJ can be done for hallux valgus correction as well as end-stage arthrosis. Two portals are used, one dorsomedially and the other plantar-medially. Lui and colleagues[7] used a 2.7-mm 30° scope, and resected the joint with an osteotome and by microfracturing the subchondral bone. Lui considered the advantages over the open technique to include better visualization, less shortening, better cosmetic results, and less postoperative pain.

CHOPART JOINT ARTHROSCOPY

While arthroscopic techniques for subtalar arthrodesis have been described in orthopedic literature since 1985, very little has been published on arthroscopic performance of calcaneocuboid and TNJ arthrodesis.[9] The only reported use of arthroscopy for midtarsal joint arthrodesis was published in 2006.[10] The midtarsal joint is approached through 4 portals: medial, dorsomedial, dorsolateral, and lateral.[19] The calcaneocuboid joint is approached through the lateral and dorsolateral portals: the lateral portal located at the plantar-lateral corner of the joint and the dorsolateral portal located in the space between the talonavicular and calcaneocuboid joints.[10] The dorsolateral portal is considered the most important portal for approach, as it exists in an area where the calcaneus, cuboid, talus, and navicular can all be visualized.[19] The talonavicular joint is approached through the medial and dorsomedial portals; with the medial portal located just dorsal to the posterior tibial tendon insertion onto the tuberosity of the navicular and the dorsomedial portal at the midpoint between the medial and dorsolateral portals.[19] Through the aforementioned portals, debridement of the articular surfaces in preparation of arthrodesis is performed prior to percutaneous placement of definitive fixation. It should be noted that there has been only one case report published on the use of arthroscopy for triple arthrodesis, which involved a post-polio equinovarus deformity that progressed to successful fusion at 4 months.[10] The use of arthroscopy for debridement of the midtarsal joint should be performed only by an experienced surgeon with excellent arthroscopic skills, and the use of cadaver limbs for fine tuning of the techniques is highly encouraged.

SUMMARY

With improved technology, and increased interest by the foot and ankle surgeon, arthroscopic treatment of small joints of the foot has become a promising tool. The 1st metatarsophalangeal joint is the most documented and refined arthroscopic approach in the small joints of the foot.[1–6,12] Various ailments of the tarsometatarsal and midtarsal joints have been treated arthroscopically, but the techniques are still being refined in comparison to the 1st MTPJ.[7–9,11] Regardless of the pathology, the surgeon must have a firm understanding of the proper anatomical considerations, indications for use, predictable outcomes, and potential complications when deciding to proceed with arthroscopic management of small joints.

REFERENCES

1. Watanabe M. Selfox-arthroscope. In: Watanabe no. 24 arthroscope (monograph). Tokyo: Teishin Hospital; 1972. p. 46–53.
2. Bartlett DH. Arthroscopic management of osteochondritis disseca. Arthroscopy 1988;4(1):51–4.
3. Debnath UK, Hemmady MV, Hariharan K. Indications for and technique of first MTP arthroscopy. Foot Ankle Int 2006;27(12):1049–54.
4. Lui TH. First metatarsophalangeal joint arthroscopy in patients with hallux valgus. Arthroscopy 2008;24(10):1122–9.
5. Wang CC, Lien SB, Huang GS, et al. Arthroscopic elimination of monosodium urate deposition of the first metatarsophalangeal joint reduces the recurrence of gout. Arthroscopy 2009;25(2):153–8.
6. Lui TH, Chan KB, Chan LK. Endoscopic distal soft-tissue release in the treatment of hallux valgus: a cadaveric study. Arthroscopy 2010;26(8):1111–6.
7. Lui TH, Chan KB, Ng S. Arthroscopic lapidus arthrodesis. Arthroscopy 2005; 21(12):1516.e1–4.
8. Lui TH. Arthroscopic tarsometatarsal (Lisfranc) arthrodesis. Knee Surg Sports Traumatol Arthrosc 2007;25:671–5.
9. Parisien JS, Vangsness T. Arthroscopy of the subtalar joint: an experimental approach. Arthroscopy 1985;1:53–7.
10. Lui TH. New technique of arthroscopic triple arthrodesis. Arthroscopy 2006;22(4): 464.e1–5.
11. Bauer T, Golano P, Hardy P. Endoscopic resection of a calcaneonavicular coalition. Knee Surg Sports Traumatol Arthrosc 2010;18:669–72.
12. Carreira DS. Arthroscopy of the hallux. Foot Ankle Clin N Am 2009;14:105–14.
13. Hirsch BE, Minugh-Purvis N. Anatomy of the lower extremity. Philadelphia: Elsevier; 2005.
14. McBride ED. The McBride bunion hallux valgus operation: refinements in the successive surgical steps of the operation. J Bone Joint Surg Am 1967;49(8): 1675–83.
15. Faure C. The skeleton of the anterior foot. Anat Clin 1981;3:49–65.
16. Shurnas PS, Coughlin MJ. Arthritic conditions of the foot. In: Coughlin MJ, Mann RA, Saltzman CL, editors. Surgery of the foot and ankle, vol. 1. 8th edition. Philadelphia: Mosby Elsevier; 2007. p. 867–906.

17. Glick JM, Ferkel RD. Arthroscopic ankle arthrodesis. In: Ferkel Richard D, editor. The foot & ankle. Philadelphia: Lippincott-Raven; 1996. p. 215–29.
18. Glick JM, Morgan CD, Myerson MS, et al. Ankle arthrodesis using an arthroscopic method: long-term follow-up of 34 cases. Arthroscopy 1996;12(4):428–34.
19. Lui TH. Arthroscopy and endoscopy of the foot and ankle: indications for new techniques. Arthroscopy 2007;23(8):889–902.

Tendoscopy of the Ankle

Jeffrey C. Christensen, DPM[a],*, Thurmond D. Lanier, DPM, MPH[b]

KEYWORDS

- Peroneus longus and brevis tendoscopy
- Posterior tibial tendoscopy • Achilles tendoscopy
- Flexor hallucis longus tendon endoscopy

Arthroscopy of the foot and ankle is a mainstream technique as a result of refined instrumentation and surgeon familiarity for a variety of pathologic conditions. With the advent of advanced arthroscopic techniques, it is a natural transition that tendoscopic techniques would be incorporated into the experienced arthroscopic surgeon's armamentarium. Tendoscopy is an endoscopy of the tendon sheath and has been described in various tendons of the foot and ankle, including the posterior tibial, peroneal, long toe flexor, anterior tibial, and Achilles tendons.[1–15] Conservative treatment of extra-articular ankle pathology is successful in most cases, but there is a 10% to 25% incidence of failed conservative treatment.[2] When conservative treatment fails, most commonly open tendon surgery is advocated. Unlike the elbow or the knee, the tendon structures of the posterior ankle are deep and can be difficult to palpate; also, these structure are in close proximity to each other, which may make diagnostic imaging challenging.[7] When treating extra-articular posterior ankle pathology, open treatment can consist of either a posterolateral or a posteromedial approach, which both imply risk of damage to adjacent structures.[2,7] Even structures that are not directly encountered during the initial dissection can become entrapped with closure of the soft tissue envelope. Surgical wound problems are of increased concern when incisions are made in the posterior ankle region. Complication rates in open surgical treatments of the Achilles tendon vary between 4.7% and 11.6% and problems are mainly wound infections, skin sloughing, and formation of painful scars.[2] With longer incisions, postoperative care may dictate the use of immobilization to promote better wound healing.[7] Tendoscopy offers the advantages of less morbidity, early range of motion, and reduction in postoperative pain.[5]

Tendoscopy of the tendons around the posterior ankle joint can be technically demanding, but can offer a unique perspective of the pathologic processes that involve these structures. There are certain anatomic constraints that can make

[a] Department of Orthopedics, Division of Podiatric Surgery, Swedish Medical Center, Seattle, WA, USA
[b] Swedish Medical Center, Seattle, WA, USA
* Corresponding author.
E-mail address: jccdpm@gmail.com

Clin Podiatr Med Surg 28 (2011) 561–570
doi:10.1016/j.cpm.2011.05.003
0891-8422/11/$ – see front matter © 2011 Elsevier Inc. All rights reserved.

tendoscopy challenging. It is imperative to understand that the lack of volume, because of advanced scarification, stenosing tenosynovitis, or confined access along the curvature of the course of a tendon, may prohibit access to the site of pathology. Furthermore, the surgeon must be aware that there is a limited view of a tendon based on the instrumentation; the light post often cannot be rotated to all positions owing to anatomic limitations of the leg. This can be even more confusing to the surgeon when scoping the peroneal tendons when it can be difficult to clearly identify which tendon is being evaluated, thus necessitating flipping the instrumentation around the tendons or using multiple portals to gain full access to the compartment.

When performing tendoscopy, the surgeon must be familiar with the anatomy of the foot and ankle. Sammarco[10] provides a solid resource of the anatomy of the peroneal tendons. Brandes and Smith[14] also provide a zonal anatomic system for the peroneal tendons. Van Dijk and Kort[5] performed a cadaveric study where they found in 3 of the 7 explorations that the peroneal tubercle on the calcaneus was between both tendons, 4 to 5 cm distal from the tip of the fibula. The posterior tibial tendon, as mentioned previously, has mesotendinous connections along its course. Van Dijk and Kort[5] offer a review of the anatomy of the posterior tibial tendon, whereas Steenstra and Van Dijk[16] provide an overview of the Achilles tendon.

Lui and colleagues[12] studied the flexor hallucis tendon and its various segments (zones). In their study, it was found that the medial plantar nerve was at the plantar medial side of the proximal tendon sheath in all specimens and its relationship to the more distal sheath was variable. Synovectomy at this location should be performed with caution because of the anatomic proximity of the tarsal tunnel structures. Therefore, any power instrumentation should be kept along the lateral aspect of the flexor hallucis longus tendon.

In this article, peroneus longus and brevis, posterior tibial, Achilles, and flexor hallucis longus tendon endoscopy are discussed individually. Tendoscopic indications and surgical technique are highlighted.

Tendoscopy developed in other anatomic regions of the body and more recently has been described in the foot and ankle. Kerr and Carpenter[17] were the first to describe arthroscopic resection of olecranon and prepatellar bursae in 6 cases. The investigators had 4 good results and 2 failures. Tendoscopy of the posterior tibial, peroneus longus and brevis, and flexor hallucis longus tendons were described by van Dijk and colleagues in 1997, 1998, and 2000 respectively.[5–7] Maquirriain[18] performed a study on 9 cadavers in which he showed that there could be adequate access to the Achilles tendon via an endoscope.

INDICATIONS/CONTRAINDICATIONS

Tendoscopy most commonly is used as a therapeutic technique, but can also be used as a diagnostic study. This can be a useful tool when imaging studies are inconclusive, especially when tendons do not take a straight course in the case of the peroneal tendons and posterior tibial tendon and increased signal intensity can be caused by the "magic angle effect."

Focal tendonitis and tenosynovitis are pathologic entities that can be treated with tendoscopy. Tenosynovitis, which is associated with chronic mechanical irritation, posttraumatic adhesions, and irregularities of the posterior aspect of the fibula or tibia, can cause significant morbidity in patients. Hypertrophy of the peroneal tubercle can cause direct repetitive injury to the peroneals as well as proximal subluxation, which can be treated with endoscopic groove deepening.[5,11] Pathologic thickening of the tissue surrounding the tendon can occur and specifically of the vincula. The vinculum is defined as mesotendinous tissue connecting tendons or tendon sheaths, which is a source of blood supply to the tendon.[19] Van Dijk and Kort[5] performed a cadaveric study where they found a consistent membranous mesotendineal structure between both peroneal tendons and tendon sheath (**Fig. 1**). This vinculum runs between the peroneus longus and peroneus brevis tendons and is attached to the posterolateral aspect of the fibula. Seven ankles in cadavers were examined by van Dijk and associates[6] where a thin vinculumlike structure was found between the posterior tibial tendon and the tendon sheath of the flexor digitorum longus. This vinculum runs all the way proximal to the end with a free edge 3 to 4 cm above the level of the posterome-dial tip of the medial malleolus. Mesotendinous thickening can become a source of morbidity, as it limits or tethers tendon excursion. This thickening can also block back-side visualization of the tendon (**Fig. 2**). Similar thickening can occur along the poste-rior tibial tendon because of overuse or stage I posterior tibial tendon dysfunction; this thickening is usually seen in the hypovascular zone posterior to the medial malleolus.[6]

Achilles tendon pathology can be classified as insertional or noninsertional entities. Insertional tendon pathology involvement is a relative contraindication for the use of tendoscopy. Likewise, wide diffuse tendinopathy remains difficult to manage with this technique. Noninsertional pathology can be divided into tendinopathy, paraten-dinopathy, and a combination of the two.[16] As discussed earlier, tendinopathy can be manifested by diffuse thickening of the tendon, local thickening, and partial tears.[16] Paratendinopathy is characterized by painful swelling around the paratenon.

SURGICAL OVERVIEW/INSTRUMENTATION

In general, tendoscopy can be performed in an outpatient setting under general, epidural, or local anesthesia. Although local anesthesia may have the disadvantage of lack of muscle relaxation, it has the distinct advantage of a dynamic examination under direct visualization.[5] This could be especially useful during peroneal tendon endoscopy to assess for tendon subluxation over the fibula or to see how the tendons function relative to the calcaneofibular ligament. The surgeon also needs to keep in mind that if hemostasis becomes an issue, the use of a thigh tourniquet may necessi-tate conversion to a general anesthetic. A thigh tourniquet is generally applied to the surgical extremity and, if needed, inflated to 120 mm Hg above mean arterial pressure.

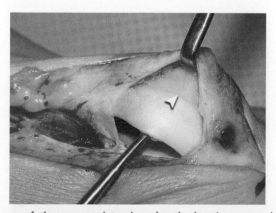

Fig. 1. Open surgery of the peroneal tendon sheath showing normal peroneus longus vinculum (*arrowhead*). Note the connection with the tendon sheath and how this would be a natural barrier for endoscopic visualization.

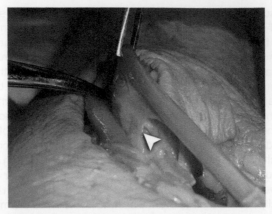

Fig. 2. Cadaver specimen depicting normal vinculum between the peroneus longus and peroneus brevis tendons. Arrowhead depicts free edge of structure.

Positioning depends on the procedure being performed and is addressed in this article when each tendon is discussed.

Standard arthroscopic equipment can be used for ankle tendoscopic procedures (**Fig. 3**). Gravity-feed or low-pressure, low-flow pump systems can be used to prevent insufflation of the subcutaneous tissue.[10] A 2.7-mm endoscope with a 30-degree tip cut is usually used when examining tendons.[2,3,5] This arthroscopic lens helps facilitate movement within the tendon sheath; the surgeon should also be cautious because this smaller-diameter scope can be more prone to breakage than larger-diameter lenses. If a significant amount of debris is anticipated (such as during a groove-deepening procedure), a 4.0-mm arthroscopic lens can be used to facilitate better flow of irrigation fluid.[3] Various instruments can be used based on the pathology visualized. Instruments such as a blunt probe, scissors, retrograde knife, and a shaver system can be used.[5]

Evaluation of the tendon pathology is the most important aspect of the procedure. Special care needs to be used to be methodical in the evaluation as well as performing a dynamic examination of tendon-gliding function (**Fig. 4**). The use of a standard

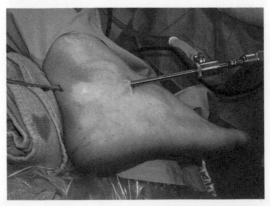

Fig. 3. Lateral position for flexor hallucis longus endoscopy using standard arthroscopic equipment. A large-diameter os trigonum was impinging on the tendon.

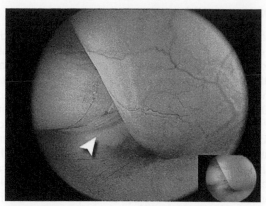

Fig. 4. Endoscopic image of distal peroneals adjacent to peroneal tubercle. Tendon gliding function was being assessed as peroneals enter separate tunnels. Note fibrous septum (*arrowhead*).

arthroscopic probe is also very effective in rotating or sliding the tendon away from the view of the scope to evaluate the back side of the tendon sheath, as well as evaluation the mesotendinous structures. Once the extent of the pathology is identified, ablative tools such as pediatric shavers/burrs, radiofrequency wands, and arthroscopic manual instrumentation are very effective in managing the pathology, especially when it involves moderate amounts of debridement of impinging types of tissue. When it comes to tendon tears (**Fig. 5**) and repairs, these conditions are variable in the surgeon's ability to fully manage with tendoscopic techniques. Open treatment may be necessary to have on the consent form, as well as tendoscopic procedures, in the event that the pathology cannot be resolved with the available instrumentation. Portals should be closed with nonabsorbable suture to prevent synovial shunt formation. The patient can usually be placed in a non–weight-bearing boot and range of motion exercises started immediately to prevent scar tissue formation and adhesions.

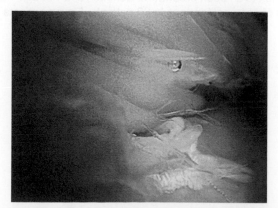

Fig. 5. Endoscopic view of partially torn and frayed peroneus brevis tendon caused by an adjacent bone spur along the fibula after fracture healing. The tendon fraying was treated with an arthroscopic shaver, whereas the bone spur required use of an arthroscopic burr. Most of the tendon was intact.

PERONEAL TENDON TENDOSCOPY

The patient is positioned on the operating room table in the lateral decubitus position with the surgical extremity up. Alternatively, the patient can be placed prone. The patient can be asked before the operation to evert the foot so the path of the tendons can be traced on the skin to be used later for portal placement. Portals can be placed anywhere along the tendon course but the 2 main portals are located directly over the tendons 1.5 to 2.0 cm distal and 2.0 to 2.5 cm proximal to the posterior edge of the lateral malleolus.[3,5] The distal portal is made first with the incision made through the skin only and blunt dissection using a hemostat is used to get through the subcutaneous tissue to avoid damage to the tendon proper to the level of the tendon sheath. The tendon sheath is penetrated by the cannula with a blunt obturator. The 2.7-mm 30-degree endoscope is then introduced into the tendon sheath. Fluid flow can then be initiated. Under direct visualization, the proximal portal can be made by introduction of a spinal needle and, once proper position of the portal is determined by the needle, the proximal portal can be made with the same technique as the distal portal was made. The most proximal portal should be made just distal to the myotendinous junction of the peroneus longus. Inspection starts 6 cm proximal from the posterior tip of the lateral malleolus where a septum splits the tendon into 2 separate compartments (see **Fig. 4**). Distally, the tendons lie in one compartment and by rotating the endoscope over and in between both tendons, the complete compartment can be inspected. Accessory portals may be made along the tendons to facilitate access to pathology, especially if an extensive synovectomy is to be performed (**Fig. 6**), or focal adhesions are identified (**Fig. 7**). An accessory portal can usually be made at the apex of the lateral malleolus to facilitate access around the curvature of the tendons. If needed, a 1.9-mm scope can be used to provide better visualization and more work space; a 70-degree scope can be helpful when working around the tip of the fibula. In cases of recurrent dislocation, fibular groove deepening can be performed. Inspection can reveal partial detachment of the superior peroneal retinaculum. The tendons can be retracted with a probe and the fibula deepened (typically 3 mm in depth and 5 mm in width) with a small burr. The burr can be introduced distally with the endoscope proximally.[11] When significant fraying or splitting is present, the tendons can become hypertrophied, which may inhibit passage of the endoscope. This will usually require a conversion to an open procedure. Scholten and van Dijk[11] described tendoscopic treatment of peroneal tendons in 23 patients. Eleven patients had longitudinal

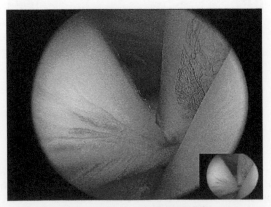

Fig. 6. Tendon endoscopy showing extensive acute synovitis.

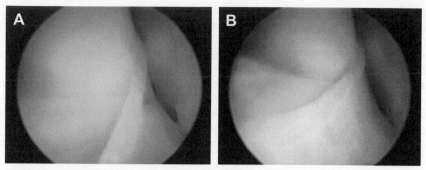

Fig. 7. (*A, B*) Images showing localized scar adhesions that wrap around the peroneus brevis like a Chinese finger trap. This occurred after tendon repair for subluxing tendons. The adhesions were severely restricting tendon excursion. Note the different orientation of same adhesions with differing foot positions. Tendon excursion was restored with adhesion resection.

rupture and were treated with a "mini-open" procedure, 10 had tenosynovitis, whereas 2 had recurrent dislocations treated with groove deepening. They reported no complications and no recurrence of preoperative pathology.

POSTERIOR TIBIAL TENDOSCOPY

The segment that is immediately distal and proximal to the medial malleolus can be accessed with tendoscopic techniques. However, this seems to require natural dilatation of the tendon sheath with the pathologic process. The patient is positioned on the operating room table in either the lateral decubitus position with the nonoperative leg up or in the supine position with the operative leg externally rotated, which can be facilitated by placing a bump under the hip of the nonoperative extremity. The course of the tendon can be marked for portal placement. The 2 main portals are located directly over the tendon 2 cm distal and 2 to 4 cm proximal to the posterior edge of the medial malleolus. Accessory portals may be placed to help in total synovectomy or to facilitate visualization around the medial malleolus. The distal portal is made first in the same manner as the peroneal tendon portals were made. Once the distal portal is made, the endoscope can be introduced into the tendon sheath and the proximal portal can be directly visualized and created. When inspecting the tendon, special attention is given to inspect the tendon sheath covering the deltoid ligament, the posterior medial malleolus surface, and the posterior ankle joint capsule.[1]

When doing posterior tibial tendon tendoscopy, there is opportunity to access the posteromedial compartment of the ankle joint. This is an advanced technique and should be practiced by surgeons who have extensive training and experience in arthroscopy. The endoscope can be introduced through the distal portal and placed between the tendon and the medial malleolus. With sagittal ankle joint motion, the joint level can be identified by palpating from the outside as well as with the probe under direct visualization from inside the tendon sheath. The obturator can then be placed in the proximal portal and used to enter the ankle joint. Synovectomy, loose body removal, or repair of a talar osteochondral lesion can then be subsequently performed.

Bulstra and colleagues[1] performed 16 procedures in 11 patients with a variety of pathology: chronic synovitis in 2, screw removal from the medial malleolus in 1, and posterior ankle arthrotomy in 2. No complications were observed. Three patients showed pathologic, thickened vincula and 4 patients showed adhesions. Two patients showed irregularity of the sliding channel, which was smoothed out. Three of the 4 patients with pathologic vincula and 2 patients who underwent tenosynovectomy and tendon release were symptom free. In general, patients did well when there was no progressive deformity. Similarly, Chow and colleagues[20] reported satisfactory endoscopic debridement of the posterior tibial tendon in stage I dysfunction in 6 patients. It should be noted that advanced pathology associated with posterior tibial insufficiency seen in adult-acquired flatfoot is a relative contraindication to the tendoscopic approach in most cases. This is because open surgery is indicated and may involve the need to advance the tendon on its insertion or perform a shortening or tendon transfer as well as the potential for major osseous procedures to augment tendon repair.

ACHILLES TENDOSCOPY

The patient is placed prone with the foot placed at the end of the table so there is full range of motion. The portals can be placed 2 cm proximal (medial to the tendon) and 2 cm distal (lateral to the tendon) to the lesion.[3,16] The distal portal is made first with an incision through the skin only. The crural fascia is penetrated by the cannula with the blunt obturator and the 2.7-mm endoscope is introduced. As in previous techniques, a spinal needle can be used to facilitate proximal portal placement.[3] In inflammatory cases, the plantaris tendon, Achilles, and paratenon are tightly bound together. Resection of the paratenon is performed on the anterior side of the tendon at the level of the painful nodule. Steenstra and Van Dijk[16] reported local resection/endoscopic release of the paratenon with no complications.

FLEXOR HALLUCIS LONGUS TENDOSCOPY

The surgical technique typically involves the posterior ankle in proximity to the posterior subtalar joint. A prone or lateral positioning allows for excellent exposure to this region (zone 1). A posterolateral portal is made at the level or slightly above the tip of the lateral malleolus, just lateral to the Achilles. A vertical incision is made and blunted down to the level of the calcaneus. A mosquito hemostat should be directed anteriorly, pointing in the direction of the interdigital web space between the first and second toe. When the tip of the hemostat touches the bone, a cannula and obturator are exchanged. A second portal can be placed anterolateral (see **Fig. 3**) or posteromedial adjacent to the Achilles tendon (prone position is preferred). The posteromedial portal is located at the same level of the posterolateral portal. After the skin incision, caution must be used when the posteromedial portal is being developed. The technique requires careful blunt dissection with a mosquito hemostat and directed laterally toward the cannula in the posterior lateral portal. This critical maneuver avoids inadvertent entry into the neurovascular bundle. The cannula is used to guide the mosquito anteriorly in the direction of the ankle/subtalar joint. The hemostat is advanced down the cannula until it touches bone. The obturator is then exchanged for the 4.0-mm lens in the posterolateral portal. The endoscope is then pulled slightly backward until the mosquito comes into view. The mosquito is used to spread the soft tissue in front of the scope. If the anterolateral portal is used, the arthroscope is placed along the lateral aspect of the posterior facet and advanced toward the posterior talus. The posterolateral portal then becomes the working portal. In cases where scar tissue or adhesions are present, a 5-mm full radius can be similarly placed and used.[7] The flexor hallucis longus tendon can then be visualized and freed of scar tissue or debrided (**Fig. 8**). Again, it is important to stay on the lateral side of the flexor hallucis longus to prevent damage to the medial neurovascular bundle.

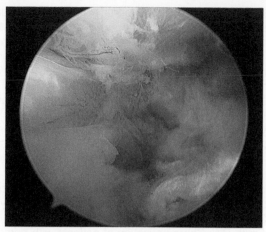

Fig. 8. Endoscopic view of the flexor hallucis longus tendon demonstrating adjacent scarification and focal acute synovitis.

SUMMARY

Hindfoot pain can be caused by a variety of pathologies, several of which can be diagnosed and treated with endoscopy. Tendoscopy of the posterior tibial, peroneal longus and brevis, Achilles, and flexor hallucis longus tendons is a useful tool to diagnose and treat focal tendon pathology. It provides a minimally invasive approach and a good alternative to the already existing open surgical approaches. Tendoscopic approaches are safe and reliable when anatomic landmarks are identified, and in combination with proper portal placement. With that being said, a relative contraindication to tendoscopy is an edematous lower extremity or extensive scarification. Results of tendoscopy of the posterior tibial, flexor hallucis longus, Achilles, and peroneal tendons seem promising as compared with open surgery, especially if there is localized pathology. Optimal portal placement for each indication has been identified in cadaveric studies. The approach for the flexor hallucis longus and os trigonum requires close attention to detail because of the adjacent neurovascular bundle. Hindfoot endoscopy gives the practitioner another treatment option for patients, and experienced arthroscopic surgeons will find this technique rewarding because of high patient satisfaction.

REFERENCES

1. Bulstra GH, Olsthoorn PG, Niek van Dijk C. Tendoscopy of the posterior tibial tendon. Foot Ankle Clin 2006;11:421–7, viii.
2. Morag G, Maman E, Arbel R. Endoscopic treatment of hindfoot pathology. Arthroscopy 2003;19:E13.
3. van Dijk CN. Hindfoot endoscopy for posterior ankle pain. Instr Course Lect 2006; 55:545–54.
4. van Dijk CN. Hindfoot endoscopy. Foot Ankle Clin 2006;11:391–414, vii.
5. van Dijk CN, Kort N. Tendoscopy of the peroneal tendons. Arthroscopy 1998;14: 471–8.
6. van Dijk CN, Kort N, Scholten PE. Tendoscopy of the posterior tibial tendon. Arthroscopy 1997;13:692–8.

7. van Dijk CN, Scholten PE, Krips R. A 2-portal endoscopic approach for diagnosis and treatment of posterior ankle pathology. Arthroscopy 2000;16:871–6.
8. Yong CK. Peroneus quartus and peroneal tendoscopy. Med J Malaysia 2006; 61(Suppl B):45–7.
9. Lui TH. Flexor hallucis longus tendoscopy: a technical note. Knee Surg Sports Traumatol Arthrosc 2009;17:107–10.
10. Sammarco VJ. Peroneal tendoscopy: indications and techniques. Sports Med Arthrosc 2009;17:94–9.
11. Scholten PE, van Dijk CN. Tendoscopy of the peroneal tendons. Foot Ankle Clin 2006;11:415–20, vii.
12. Lui TH, Chan KB, Chan LK. Cadaveric study of zone 2 flexor hallucis longus tendon sheath. Arthroscopy 2010;26(6):808–12.
13. Frey C. Surgical advancements: arthroscopic alternatives to open procedures: great toe, subtalar joint, Haglund's deformity and tendoscopy. Foot Ankle Clin 2009;14:313–39.
14. Brandes CB, Smith RW. Characterization of patients with primary peroneus longus tendinopathy: a review of twenty-two cases. Foot Ankle Int 2000;212:462–8.
15. Lui TH, Chan BK, Chan LK. Zone 2 flexor hallucis longus tendoscopy: a cadaveric study. Foot Ankle Int 2009;30:447–51.
16. Steenstra F, Van Dijk CV. Achilles tendoscopy. Foot Ankle Clin 2006;11:429–38.
17. Kerr DR, Carpenter CW. Arthroscopic resection of olecranon and prepatellar bursae. Arthroscopy 1990;6(2):86–8.
18. Maquirriain J. Endoscopic release of Achilles peritenon. Arthroscopy 1998;14(2): 182–5.
19. Sarrafian SK. Anatomy of the foot and ankle: descriptive, topographic, and functional. 2nd edition. Philadelphia: Lippincott; 1993.
20. Chow HT, Chan BK, Lui TH. Tendoscopic debridement for stage I posterior tibial tendon dysfunction. Knee Surg Sports Traumatol Arthrosc 2005;13:695–8.

Current Concepts and Techniques in Foot and Ankle Surgery

Antithrombotic Pharmacologic Prophylaxis Use During Conservative and Surgical Management of Foot and Ankle Disorders: A Systematic Review

Valerie L. Schade, DPM, AACFAS[a],*, Thomas S. Roukis, DPM, PhD[b]

KEYWORDS

• Deep venous thrombosis • Low molecular weight heparin
• Pulmonary embolism • Venous thromboembolism

There are currently no widely accepted standardized guidelines regarding the use of antithrombotic pharmacologic prophylaxis during conservative or postoperative management of foot and ankle disorders. Recommendations range from providing antithrombotic pharmacologic prophylaxis to high-risk patients only to providing no prophylaxis at all based on the low reported incidence of clinically significant deep venous thrombosis (DVT) and pulmonary embolus (PE) associated with conservative or postoperative management of foot and ankle disorders.[1–16] The current guidelines from the American College of Chest Physicians (ACCP) are not specific to foot and ankle disorders and instead address isolated injuries of the lower extremity, defined as any tendinous or osseous injury occurring distal to the knee.[17] In this guideline,

---

Disclaimer: the opinions or assertions contained herein are the private view of the author and are not to be construed as official or reflecting the views of the Department of the Army or the Department of Defense.

The authors have nothing to disclose and have no conflict of interest to report.

[a] Limb Preservation Service, Vascular/Endovascular Surgery Service, Department of Surgery, Madigan Healthcare System, 9040 Fitzsimmons Drive, MCHJ-SV, Tacoma, WA 98431, USA
[b] Department of Orthopaedics, Podiatry, and Sports Medicine, Gundersen Lutheran Medical Center, 2nd Floor Founder's Building, 1900 South Avenue, La Crosse, WI 54601, USA
* Corresponding author.
E-mail address: vlsdpm@gmail.com

Clin Podiatr Med Surg 28 (2011) 571–588
doi:10.1016/j.cpm.2011.04.004
0891-8422/11/$ – see front matter. Published by Elsevier Inc.

podiatric.theclinics.com

data were reviewed from 6 randomized clinical trials, 2 focused on conservative management of lower extremities injuries and the incidence of DVT/PE and 4 focused on the postoperative management of below-knee fracture open reduction and internal fixation (ORIF) and surgical repair of Achilles tendon rupture and the incidence of DVT/PE. The pooled data demonstrated that patients with lower extremity injuries had a 10% to 45% risk of developing an asymptomatic DVT. Risk factors associated with the development of DVT/PE were found to be older age, surgical intervention, obesity, fractures, and Achilles tendon ruptures. The use of low molecular weight heparin (LMWH) was found to reduce the frequency of asymptomatic DVT, particularly in cases of surgical repair of Achilles tendon rupture. However, as these trials only addressed asymptomatic DVT/PE, it was determined that the results could not be extrapolated to clinically significant DVT/PE. The cost-effectiveness of providing antithrombotic pharmacologic prophylaxis for isolated lower extremity injuries was not reported. Based on these considerations, the ACCP does not currently recommend the use of routine antithrombotic pharmacologic prophylaxis for injuries of the lower extremity distal to the knee.

This is in contrast with the current protocol of the authors that involves administration of antithrombotic pharmacologic prophylaxis in the form of a weight-based prophylactic dose of heparin (5000 international units twice or 3 times a day) while patients are hospitalized and the use of a prophylactic dose of LMWH (40 mg Lovenox once daily) on discharge, which is administered until the patient is fully ambulatory. The use of mechanical prophylaxis in the form of sequential compression devices is also used while patients are hospitalized, and compression stockings for the contralateral limb during the recovery period. All patients treated by the authors are considered moderate to high risk because of the presence of evidenced-based risk factors for the development of DVT/PE including advanced age, increased body weight, presence of varicose veins, and after lower extremity surgery being performed under general anesthesia (**Box 1**).[18–20] Despite the use of pharmacologic and mechanical antithrombotic prophylaxis, the authors have experienced the formation of DVT leading to PE, which was a near-fatal event in 1 patient and a fatal event in another.[21] Given our standard protocol for antithrombotic pharmacologic and mechanical prophylaxis and the controversy that remains regarding administration of antithrombotic pharmacologic prophylaxis during treatment of foot and ankle disorders, a systematic review was undertaken to determine the incidence of DVT/PE during conservative or postoperative management of traumatic injuries or elective surgery of the foot and ankle in patients who did or did not receive antithrombotic pharmacologic prophylaxis for any portion of the recovery period, as well as to determine whether antithrombotic pharmacologic prophylaxis reduces the incidence of either asymptomatic or symptomatic DVT/PE.

MATERIALS AND METHODS

Eleven electronic databases, including the American College of Physicians Journal Club (http://www.acpjc.org/), Cumulative Index of Nursing and Allied Health Literature (http://www.ebscohost.com/cinahl/), Cochrane Collaboration Library (http://www.thecochranelibrary.com/view/0/index.html?CRETRY&;), Cochrane Controlled Trials Register (http://www.ovid.com/site/products/ovidguide/cctrdb.htm), The Cochrane Collaboration Cochrane Reviews (http://www.cochrane.org/reviews/), Cochrane Methodology Register (cmr.cochrane.org), Center for Reviews and Dissemination (http://www.crd.york.ac.uk/crdweb/Home.aspx?DB=DARE), The Cochrane Library (http://mrw.interscience.wiley.com/cochrane/cochrane_clhta_articles_fs.html), Infotrieve-PubMed/MEDLINE (http://www4.infotrieve.com/newmedline/search.asp),

Box 1
Risk factors for postoperative DVT

- Risk Factors
  o **Age**
  o **Obesity**
  o **Past history of DVT/PE**
  o **Tobacco use**
  o **Varicose veins**
  o Pregnancy
  o **Oral contraceptive use**
  o Hormone replacement therapy
  o Female
  o Ethnicity/race
  o **Malignancy**
  o Chemotherapy
  o Thrombophilia
  o **Factor V Leiden mutation**
  o Cardiovascular factors
  o Type of anesthesia: **general**
  o Type of surgery: **orthopaedic**

Risk factors with evidence showing a significant association are in bold type.

Data from Refs.[18–20]

and Ovid MEDLINE(R) In-Process and other nonindexed citations (http://www.ovid.com/site/products/ovidguide/medline.htm) were searched from inception to July 2010. The search was restricted to the English language with no restriction on date using an inclusive text word query for "foot" AND "ankle" AND "immobilization" OR "cast" OR "orthosis" AND "surgical" OR "nonsurgical" AND "deep venous thrombosis" OR "pulmonary embolism" OR "thromboembolism" AND "prophylaxis" OR "thromboprophylaxis" OR "low molecular weight heparin" with the words in all upper case representing the Boolean operators used. To maximize the number of potentially useful references, every combination of text words was queried through each of the electronic databases. In addition, an Internet-based general interest search engine, specifically Google (http://www.google.com/), was used to identify available sources that could potentially provide useful information, by using various combinations of the text words listed earlier. References from each manuscript identified were hand searched to identify any pertinent material for review that was not identified from the electronic searches. If a reference could not be obtained through purchase, librarian assistance, or email contact with the author, it was excluded from consideration. Studies were eligible for inclusion if they were prospective studies, randomized or nonrandomized, with consecutive enrollment of subjects undergoing conservative treatment or postoperative management of traumatic injuries or elective surgery of foot and ankle disorders that received either antithrombotic pharmacologic prophylaxis for any portion of the treatment period, placebo, or were untreated for thrombotic events. Diagnosis of DVT had to have objective confirmation with either duplex ultrasonography (DUS) showing a noncompressible lumen or ascending phlebography showing a segment-filling defect on 1 or more views. A proximal DVT was defined as a thrombosis occurring within or proximal to the popliteal vein. A distal DVT was defined as a thrombosis occurring distal to the popliteal vein. The diagnosis of PE had to have objective confirmation with either a computed tomography pulmonary angiogram or ventilation/perfusion scan for inclusion in analysis (**Box 2**). The incidence of major or minor bleeding complications was assessed when reported but was not a requirement for inclusion in analysis.

RESULTS

The search for potentially eligible information for inclusion in the systematic review yielded a total of 36 publications. All publications were obtained and reviewed in their entirety by the authors in July 2010. On completion of review, 15 publications were determined potentially eligible for inclusion in analysis.[22–36] Detailed review of these references revealed that 1 reference was a quasi-systematic review, 1 reference was a meta-analysis with different study inclusion parameters, and 1 reference was a response to another study for further clarification of the data presented in the study.[22–24,30] In addition, 4 references did not meet the inclusion criteria because of the inability to determine whether the trauma sustained was localized to the foot and ankle or included injuries of the proximal lower leg (ie, tibial plateau fractures).[25,27,30,36] This left 8 publications (22.2%) that met all the inclusion criteria.[26,28,29,31–35] Three were related to the use of antithrombotic pharmacologic prophylaxis during conservative management of traumatic foot and ankle injuries and 5 were related to the use of antithrombotic pharmacologic prophylaxis during the postoperative management of elective surgery and surgical repair of traumatic foot and ankle injuries (**Tables 1** and **2**).

Box 2
Inclusion criteria

- Prospective, randomized, or nonrandomized study
- Consecutive enrollment of patients
- Conservative or postoperative management of:
  - Traumatic injuries restricted to the foot and/or ankle
  - Elective surgery of disorders restricted to the foot and/or ankle
- Patients received either:
  - No antithrombotic pharmacologic prophylaxis
  - Placebo
  - Any type of antithrombotic pharmacologic prophylaxis of any duration during the treatment period
- DVT confirmed with either:
  - Duplex ultrasonography (DUS) showing a noncompressible lumen
  - Ascending phlebography showing a segment filling on 1 or more views
- PE confirmed with either:
  - Computed tomography pulmonary angiogram
  - Ventilation/perfusion scan

Table 1
Conservative management

Author, Year	Study Type (Level of Evidence)	MOI	Patients Screened	Total Number of Patients	Male	Female	Mean Age (y)	Number Receiving Prophylaxis (%)	Mean Time of Immobilization (d)	DVT (%)	PE (%)	Time to Diagnosis DVT/PE (d)
Kock et al,[26] 1995	Prospective, randomized, single center (level 1, therapeutic)	Trauma	All	339	208	131	34	176 (51.9)	14	5 (1.5)	0 (0)	11
Patil et al,[32] 2007	Prospective, single center (level 2, therapeutic)	Trauma	All	100	51	49	43	None (0)	42	5 (5.0)	0 (0)	42
Riou et al,[34] 2007	Prospective, observational, multicenter (level 2, therapeutic)	Trauma	All	2739	1391	1358	40	1680 (61.1)	22	177 (6.5)	1 (0.04)	22

Abbreviation: MOI, mechanism of injury.

Table 2
Postoperative management

Author, Year	Study Type (Level of Evidence)	Reason for Surgery	Patients Screened	Total Number of Patients	Male	Female	Mean Age (y)	Number Receiving Prophylaxis (%)	Mean Time of Immobilization (d)	DVT (%)	PE (%)	Time to Diagnosis DVT/PE (d)
Mizel et al,[31] 1998	Prospective, multicenter (level 2, therapeutic)	Elective and trauma	Symptomatic only	2733	1027	1706	48	2504 (91.6)	NS	6 (0.22)	4 (0.15)	35
Solis and Saxby,[35] 2002	Prospective, single center (level 2, therapeutic)	Elective and trauma	All	201	83	118	46	0 (0)	NS	7 (3.5)	0 (0)	11
Radl et al,[33] 2003	Prospective, single center (level 2, therapeutic)	Hallux valgus Elective surgery	All	100	9	91	49	0 (0)	0	4 (4.0)	0 (0)	29
Lapidus et al,[28] 2007	Prospective, randomized, placebo-controlled, single center (level 1, therapeutic)	Ankle fracture ORIF	All	226*	UN	UN	49	101 (44.7)	44	58 (25.7)	0 (0)	44
Lapidus et al,[29] 2007	Prospective, randomized, placebo-controlled, single center (level 1, therapeutic)	Achilles tendon rupture repair	All	96*	UN	UN	40	49 (51.0)	43	37 38.5	0 (0)	28

Abbreviations: NS, not stated; UN, unknown.
* Total number of patients who underwent DVT surveillance.

CONSERVATIVE TREATMENT

There were a total of 339 patients in the study by Kock and colleagues,[26] with 176 patients receiving 32 mg LMWH (specific medication not stated) daily by subcutaneous injection and the remaining 163 patients being untreated (see **Table 1**). The duration of antithrombotic pharmacologic prophylaxis was not mentioned. Injuries were classified as grade II strains and bruises, grade III strains, fractures, or others. All were treated with a below-knee cast with weight-bearing status not mentioned. The mean immobilization time was 11 (range 1–29) days in the treatment group and 17 (range 1–76) days in the untreated control. All patients were screened using DUS for DVT at the time of cast removal. All DVT diagnosed with DUS were confirmed with ascending phlebography. Although the injuries could not be specifically localized to the foot and ankle, 5 of the 7 DVT reported occurred in patients who sustained trauma to the foot or ankle (ie, 1 fracture of the hallux, 1 fracture of the fifth metatarsal, 1 contusion of the ankle, 1 tear of an ankle ligament, and 1 severe distortion of the ankle). All DVT occurred in the untreated control group. Of these 5 DVT, 2 were proximal and 3 were distal. Proximal DVT occurred in the patients who sustained the fracture of the hallux and the tear of an ankle ligament. It was not stated whether any of the DVT were symptomatic. No PE were reported. The mean age of the patients with a DVT was 55 (±6.7) years (range, 47–60 years). The mean time to diagnosis of DVT was 11 (range 1–29) days. All DVT occurred in patients greater or equal to 40 years old in below-knee cast immobilization, with some patients having undergone immobilization for less then 10 days. There were no major bleeding complications reported. Five minor complications were reported consisting of 4 small local hematomas at the injection site and 1 incidence of facial eczema.

The study by Patil and colleagues[32] focused on conservative treatment of ankle fractures with cast immobilization (see **Table 1**). The mean time of immobilization was 42 (range 21–49) days, which was the longest mean immobilization time of all 3 studies included in our systematic review of conservative treatment of traumatic injuries of the foot and ankle. None of the patients received antithrombotic pharmacologic prophylaxis. All patients were screened for DVT using DUS at the time of cast removal. A total of 5 DVT occurred with 3 being distal and 2 being proximal. All DVT were asymptomatic. There was no PE reported. The mean age of those who developed a DVT was 50 (range 18–69) years. Four of the 5 patients had a body mass index (BMI) greater than 28. Three of the 5 patients had a current tobacco use history. All patients with a DVT were allowed to bear full weight in their cast during treatment. No minor or major bleeding complications were reported.

Riou and colleagues[34] provide the largest number of patients in their prospective, multicenter observational study (see **Table 1**). Administration of antithrombotic pharmacologic prophylaxis was not standardized but based on the discretion of the treating emergency room physician due to the concern for potential development of DVT/PE. The 4 risk factors found to be the most influential for prompting the treating emergency room physician to start antithrombotic pharmacologic prophylaxis was the need for cast immobilization, the requirement for non–weight-bearing, and severe or moderate injury. A total of 1680 patients received antithrombotic pharmacologic prophylaxis (specific medication not stated), and 1059 patients received no prophylaxis. As administration of antithrombotic pharmacological prophylaxis was at the discretion of the treating emergency room physician and not standardized, the type prescribed was not reported. Antithrombotic pharmacologic prophylaxis continued for the entire period of immobilization with a mean immobilization time of 22 days. All patients were screened for DVT using DUS on completion of their immobilization period. There were a total of 177 (6.4%) DVT reported with 172 being distal and 5 being proximal. One DVT progressed to a PE (0.04%). There were 27 (15.3%) symptomatic DVT. The study found that the risk factors prompting antithrombotic pharmacologic prophylaxis were accurate for predicting patients at high risk for developing DVT/PE. Age greater than 50 years was found to be an additional risk factor for the potential to develop DVT/PE. Obesity, previous history of DVT/PE, family history of DVT/PE, and malignancy could not be assessed as potential risk factors for DVT/PE because of the small proportion of patients with these factors included in the study. The study could not assess the protective role of antithrombotic pharmacologic prophylaxis; however, the investigators believed that the role of antithrombotic pharmacologic prophylaxis was favorable because of the low reported incidence of DVT/PE. No minor or major bleeding complications were reported; however, the investigators stated that complications related to the use of antithrombotic pharmacologic prophylaxis were low and not usually severe. The investigators suggested that the risk-versus-benefit potential weighted favorably for the use of antithrombotic pharmacologic prophylaxis.

The weighted data for all 3 studies involving conservative management of traumatic foot and ankle injuries included 3188 patients (1650 men and 1538 women), with 1856 (58.2%) receiving some type of antithrombotic pharmacologic prophylaxis and 1332 (41.8%) receiving no prophylaxis during their conservative treatment period. The weighted mean age was 39 years and the weighted mean time of immobilization was 22 days. The total incidence of DVT was 187 (5.9%) and PE was 1 (0.03%). Of the 187 DVT reported, 178 (95.2%) were distal and 9 (4.8%) were proximal, with 27 (14.4%) of the DVT being symptomatic. The weighted mean time to diagnosis of DVT/PE was 22 days. The risk factors found to have a strong association with the occurrence of DVT/PE were age greater than 40 years, immobilization with or without a cast, obesity, and severe injury.

POSTOPERATIVE MANAGEMENT

Mizel and colleagues[31] had the study with the largest number of patients (2733) of all the studies included in our systematic review (see **Table 2**). This study had consecutive enrollment of all patients undergoing elective surgery or surgical repair of traumatic foot and ankle injuries. The data on patients with subsequent DVT/PE were not categorized between those patients who underwent elective surgery or surgical repair of a traumatic injury. All traumatic injuries were isolated injuries of the foot and ankle. The only exclusion criterion for the study was multiple traumatic injuries. A total of 2504 (91.6%) patients received some form of antithrombotic pharmacologic prophylaxis, and 229 (8.4%) patients received no prophylaxis. The type of antithrombotic pharmacologic prophylaxis administered, the reason for administration, and the duration of prophylaxis were not stated. Only patients with clinical symptoms concerning for DVT or PE were screened. A diagnosis of DVT was confirmed with either DUS or ascending phlebography, and PE was confirmed with ventilation and perfusion scans. The mean time to diagnosis of DVT was 35 days. There were a total of 6 (0.22%) DVTs reported, with 4 being distal and 2 being proximal. Four (0.15%) DVTs, 2 distal and 2 proximal, progressed to PE. The study found that the risk factors associated with an increased incidence of DVT/PE were non–weight-bearing requirement, and immobilization. There was no relationship found with age, weight, history of previous DVT/PE, malignancy, diabetes, cardiac disease, hypertension, tourniquet use, site of tourniquet application, duration of tourniquet use, harvest of iliac crest bone graft, arthrodesis, open reduction of fractures with internal fixation, or soft tissue or osseous surgery. No minor or major bleeding complications were reported.

The study by Solis and Saxby[35] also involved the consecutive enrollment of all patients undergoing elective surgery or surgical repair of traumatic foot and ankle injuries (see **Table 2**). All patients in the study were screened for DVT with DUS at their first postoperative appointment, which was at a mean of 11 (range 6–18) days. Patients excluded in the study were those who did not make their first postoperative appointment, those on anticoagulant therapy before surgery, and those with a previous history of DVT/PE, because it is routine practice by the investigators of the study to give prophylaxis to these patients. The type of antithrombotic pharmacologic prophylaxis administered, the reason for administration, and the duration of prophylaxis was not stated. Those patients who had a distal DVT identified at their first postoperative appointment had a repeat DUS 1 week later to determine whether the DVT had progressed proximally. Progression was not seen with any of the distal DVT identified in the study. A total of 7 (3.5%) DVT were identified. All DVT were distal, with 5 being completely occlusive and 2 being nonocclusive. All of the DVT were asymptomatic. There was no PE reported. There were 4 risk factors found to have an association with development of nonocclusive and occlusive DVT. These risk factors were immobilization, hindfoot surgery with and without immobilization, and obesity. Age and increased tourniquet time had a significant association with nonocclusive DVT only. No minor or major bleeding complications were reported.

Radl and colleagues[33] focused on the incidence of DVT after a chevron osteotomy for hallux valgus correction (see **Table 2**). Patients were allowed to be fully weight bearing in a stiff-soled shoe immediately after surgery and were instructed to perform ankle dorsiflexion and plantarflexion several times per day after surgery. All patients underwent a unilateral ascending phlebography an average of 29 days after surgery. A total of 4 (4%) DVT were identified. All DVT were distal and asymptomatic. There were no PE reported. There was no association found between obesity, duration of surgery, and oral contraceptive use/hormone replacement therapy use and the development of DVT. Age greater than 60 years was found to have a strong association with the development of DVT. No minor or major bleeding complications were reported.

Lapidus and colleagues[28,29] performed 2 randomized, placebo-controlled, double-blind studies (see **Table 2**). The first study reported on the use of prolonged antithrombotic pharmacologic prophylaxis after ORIF of ankle fractures.[28] Dalteparin 5000 international units administered daily via subcutaneous injection was given for a total of 7 days to all patients in both the treatment and placebo-controlled group. The treatment group then continued with this for the duration of immobilization, whereas the placebo-controlled group received 9% sodium chloride in identical prefilled syringes. There were a total of 136 patients each in the treatment and placebo-controlled groups. One patient in the placebo group developed a DVT prior to the start of the study and was excluded. Thirty five patients in the treatment group and 39 patients in the placebo group were lost to follow up. A total of 101 patients in the treatment group and 96 patients in the placebo group underwent DVT surveillance. On removal of cast immobilization, all patients were screened for DVT with unilateral ascending phlebography. DUS was used when phlebography could not be performed because of failure to obtain venous access. The mean immobilization time was 44 days with the mean time of antithrombotic pharmacologic prophylaxis administered being 35 days in the treatment group. A total of 24 (24.7%) DVT occurred in the treatment group, with 20 being distal and 4 being proximal. A total of 34 (27.2%) DVT occurred in the placebo-controlled group, with 31 being distal and 3 being proximal. Of those with DVT, 18 (13.2%) in the treatment group were immobilized in a cast compared with 27 (19.9%) in the control group. There was no

PE reported in either group. Of all the DVT, 8 (13.8%) were symptomatic, with 2 occurring in the treatment group and 6 occurring in the placebo-controlled group. Of the 8 symptomatic DVT, 1 was proximal, 6 were distal and 1 was in a muscular vein. The only risk factor found to have a strong association with development of DVT/PE was cast immobilization. The potential for DVT/PE with the use of cast immobilization was found to be significantly reduced with prolonged antithrombotic pharmacologic prophylaxis. No major bleeding complications were reported. One minor bleed occurred in both the treatment and placebo-controlled groups. Treatment was discontinued for both of these patients, with 1 subsequently developing a symptomatic DVT. It was not reported whether this patient had been in the treatment or the placebo-controlled group.

The second study by Lapidus and colleagues[29] reported on the use of prolonged antithrombotic pharmacologic prophylaxis after surgical repair of Achilles tendon ruptures (see **Table 2**). Dalteparin 5000 international units daily via subcutaneous injection was given to the treatment group for the duration of immobilization, whereas the placebo-controlled group received 9% sodium chloride in identical prefilled syringes. It was not stated whether both groups received this for the initial postoperative week as was performed in the previous study. There were a total of 52 patients in the treatment group and 53 patients in the placebo-controlled group with 2 patients lost to follow up in each group. A total of 49 patients in the treatment group and 47 patients in the placebo group underwent DVT surveillance. On removal of cast immobilization all patients were screened for DVT with DUS. All DVT found with DUS was confirmed with unilateral phlebography. The mean time to diagnosis of DVT was 28 days. A total of 18 (36.7%) DVT occurred in the treatment group, with 17 being distal and 1 being proximal. A total of 19 (40.4%) DVT occurred in the placebo-controlled group, with 16 being distal and 3 being proximal. There was no PE reported in either group. No major bleeding complications were reported. There was 1 minor bleed in the treatment group only. Treatment was discontinued and this patient subsequently developed a DVT 14 days later. The study did not report the number of symptomatic DVT occurring in either the treatment or the placebo-controlled group because of the inability to differentiate normal postoperative pain from calf pain likely related to DVT. Although no risk factors were specifically reported to have a strong association with development of DVT/PE, the investigators believed it prudent to provide antithrombotic pharmacologic prophylaxis for patients requiring surgical repair of Achilles tendon ruptures with subsequent immobilization.

The weighted data reported for all 5 studies involving postoperative management of elective surgery or surgical repair of traumatic foot and ankle injuries involved 3356 patients who underwent DVT surveillance. The gender of the subjects who underwent DVT surveillance could not be determine in two studies.[28,29] Of the remaining studies, there were 1119 men and 1915 women. A total of 2654 (79.1%) patients received some type of antithrombotic pharmacologic prophylaxis and 702 (20.9%) received either no prophylaxis or placebo during their postoperative management. There were 10 (0.29%) patients in whom it was unknown whether or not antithrombotic pharmacologic prophylaxis was administered. The weighted mean age was 48 years. The total incidence of DVT was 112 (3.3%) and of PE was 4 (0.12%). Of the 112 DVT reported, 99 (88.4%) were distal and 11 (11.6%) were proximal, with 14 (12.5%) DVT being symptomatic. The weighted mean time to diagnosis of DVT/PE was 36 days. The risk factors found to have a strong association for the occurrence of DVT/PE were age greater than 40 years, immobilization, non–weight-bearing requirement, hindfoot surgery with or without immobilization, obesity, and increased tourniquet time.

DISCUSSION

The purpose of this systematic review was to evaluate the best evidence available for determining the incidence of DVT/PE during conservative or postoperative management of traumatic injuries or elective surgery of the foot and ankle in patients who did or did not receive antithrombotic pharmacologic prophylaxis of any type and any duration during the recovery period, and to determine whether antithrombotic pharmacologic prophylaxis reduces the incidence of DVT/PE. The systematic review was performed according to the well-described principles of performing systematic reviews.[37] Of the 36 publications identified, 8 (22.2%) met all of our inclusion criteria.[26,28,29,31–35] The included studies were of good to high methodological design (level I or II therapeutic studies).

Most DVT diagnosed in both the conservative and postoperative treatment groups were distal rather than proximal: 95.2% in the conservative management group and 88.4% in the postoperative management group. This finding is consistent with the known natural history of DVT.[38] Distal DVT has been reported to have a propagation rate ranging from 5.6% to 32% in postoperative patients.[39–41] The risk for proximal progression of distal DVT also increases with the continued presence of risk factors for DVT, such as continued immobilization.[38] Most DVT in both groups were also asymptomatic: 85.6% in the conservative management group and 92.9% in the postoperative management group. Lapidus and colleagues[29] considered that the classic signs of DVT (ie, unilateral swelling and calf pain) may not be useful in creating an increased index of suspicion for DVT in patients who have undergone surgery involving the foot and ankle because of the normal postoperative recovery course, which entails pain and swelling of the lower extremity. Although the primary concern in preventing DVT is the reduction of mortality related to PE, preventing DVT may also aid in the long-term morbidity associated with postthrombotic syndrome (PTS).[42,43] PTS develops because of the damage to venous valves or outflow obstruction related to the DVT.[44] This potential long-term consequence of DVT can result in chronic pain, chronic swelling, eczema, and ulcerations that can develop months or years after initial development of DVT.[42,44–46] A meta-analysis of PTS related to asymptomatic DVT revealed that there is an increased incidence of PTS.[46] PTS has been shown to be up to 16% in patients diagnosed with a distal DVT up to 2 years later, with the severity of symptoms worsening with increasing time from the initial DVT diagnosis.[38,42,46] PTS in multiple calf veins, as opposed to a single calf vein, has also been reported to result in a more frequent and severe incidence of PTS.[43] The long-term fiscal burden specific to treatment of subsequent venous leg ulceration has been estimated to be $1 billion dollars in the United States. Thus, the use of antithrombotic pharmacologic prophylaxis to prevent DVT may be justified not only on the clinical grounds of protection against a fatal PE but the initial cost may outweigh the long-term fiscal burden presented with treatment of the long-term complications of PTS.[42,46] Willie-Jørgensen and colleagues[46] reported an 8% overall risk reduction of PTS with a number needed to treat of 13 asymptomatic postoperative DVT to prevent 1 case of PTS.

The cost of antithrombotic pharmacologic prophylaxis related to the treatment of minor or major bleeding complications also seems to be negligible. The rate of bleeding complications was not reported in every study involving conservative or postoperative management of the foot and ankle. However, in those studies in which these complications were reported, they were only related to minor bleeding events. No major bleeding complications were reported. Leonardi and colleagues[47] performed a systematic review of 33 randomized controlled trials regarding the rate of bleeding complications after antithrombotic pharmacologic prophylaxis. The incidence of minor bleeding complications was found to be low: injection site bleeding, 6.9%; wound hematoma, 5.7%; drain site bleeding, 2.0%; and hematuria, 1.6%. The incidence of major bleeding complications was still lower: gastrointestinal bleed, 0.2% and retroperitoneal bleed, 0.08%. The need for operation related to bleeding complications was the same as that found with placebo at 0.7%. The incidence of discontinuation of antithrombotic pharmacologic prophylaxis was only 2.0%. Injection site bruising and wound hematomas were the 2 most common complications and were found to be higher in those receiving antithrombotic pharmacologic prophylaxis requiring multiple daily injections. Discontinuation of antithrombotic pharmacologic prophylaxis was also higher in those requiring multiple daily injections. Although the impact of pain associated with daily injections was not evaluated, the overall findings from the study show that both minor and major bleeding complications related to the administration of antithrombotic pharmacologic prophylaxis are low. Compliance with self administration of antithrombotic pharmacologic prophylaxis has also been found to be good to excellent with proper patient education on the necessity of its use.[48]

Reviewing the combined data for the studies included in our systematic review, the number of patients in both the conservative and postoperative management groups was equivalent. The total reported incidence of DVT/PE in both the conservative and postoperative management groups was low: 5.9% DVT and 0.03% PE, and 3.3% DVT and 0.12% PE respectively. However, more than half of the patients received some type of antithrombotic pharmacologic prophylaxis for some portion of the treatment period (58.2% and 79.1% respectively). The incidence of DVT/PE for patients who received any form of antithrombotic pharmacologic prophylaxis for any duration of the treatment period cannot be adequately determined in those studies involving conservative management of disorders affecting the foot and ankle. Of the 187 DVT and 1 PE reported, 177 DVT and the 1 PE were reported in the study by Riou and colleagues,[34] who did not state whether these patients received antithrombotic pharmacologic prophylaxis (**Table 3**).

The incidence of DVT/PE for those patients who did receive some form of antithrombotic pharmacologic prophylaxis for some portion of the treatment period is more telling in the studies involving postoperative management of disorders affecting the foot and ankle. Only 1 study did not state whether those patients with DVT (6) or PE (4) received antithrombotic pharmacologic prophylaxis. Of the remaining 106 DVT reported, 64 (60.4%) occurred in patients who received no antithrombotic pharmacologic prophylaxis, compared with 42 (39.6%) who received Dalteparin 5000 units daily for the length of immobilization (mean 36 days) (**Table 4**). The only 2 randomized, placebo-controlled, double-blind studies included in the analysis were in the postoperative management group, with both studies finding that the potential for DVT/PE during postoperative management of disorders affecting the foot and ankle was significantly reduced with prolonged antithrombotic pharmacologic prophylaxis, particularly after surgical repair of a ruptured Achilles tendon.[28,29]

In addition, most of the studies excluded patients with known risk factors for the development of DVT/PE: listed from most to least frequently excluded risk factors: previous history of DVT or PE, varicose veins, chronic venous insufficiency, prior lower extremity vein surgery, immobilization, trauma occurring greater or equal to 48 hours before presentation, and malignancy.[26,28,29,33–35] The highest incidence of DVT in the conservative management group occurred in the study in which patients were prescribed antithrombotic pharmacologic prophylaxis based on the emergency room physician's concern that these patients were at high risk for development of DVT/PE.[34] These findings support the concern that certain factors place patients at

Table 3
Conservative management DVT/PE reported in patients who did and did not receive antithrombotic pharmacologic prophylaxis

Author, Year	Total Number of Patients	Number Receiving Prophylaxis (%)	Number Receiving No Prophylaxis (%)	ATTP Type	ATTP Duration (d)	Total DVT (%)	DVT ATTP (%)	DVT No ATTP (%)	Total PE (%)	PE ATTP (%)	PE No ATTP (%)
Kock et al,[26] 1995	339	176 (51.9)	163 (48.1)	32 mg LWMH daily[a]	NS	5 (1.5)	0 (0)	5 (1.5)	0 (0)	0 (0)	0 (0)
Patil et al,[32] 2007	100	None (0)	100 (100)	None	NA	5 (5.0)	0 (0)	5 (5.0)	0 (0)	0 (0)	0 (0)
Riou et al,[34] 2007	2739	1680 (61.3)	1059 (38.7)	UN	22[b]	177 (6.5)	UN	UN	1 (0.04)	UN	UN

Abbreviations: ATTP, antithrombotic pharmacologic prophylaxis; NA, not applicable; NS, not stated; UN, unknown.
[a] Type of ATTP not stated.
[b] Mean duration of immobilization.

Table 4
Postoperative management DVT/PE reported in patients who did and did not receive antithrombotic pharmacologic prophylaxis

Author, Year	Total Number of Patients	Number Receiving Prophylaxis (%)	Number Receiving No Prophylaxis (%)	ATTP Type	ATTP Duration (d)	Total DVT (%)	DVT ATTP (%)	DVT No ATTP (%)	Total PE (%)	PE ATTP (%)	PE No ATTP (%)
Mizel et al,[31] 1998	2733	2504 (91.6)	229 (8.4)	NS	NS	6 (0.22)	UN	UN	4 (0.15)	UN	UN
Solis and Saxby,[35] 2002	201	0 (0)	201 (100)	None	NA	7 (3.5)	0 (0)	7 (3.5)	0 (0)	0 (0)	0 (0)
Radl et al,[33] 2003	100	0 (0)	100 (100)	None	NA	4 (4.0)	0 (0)	4 (4.0)	0 (0)	0 (0)	0 (0)
Lapidus et al,[28] 2007	226*	101 (44.7)	125 (55.3)	Dalteparin 5000 units daily[a]	44[b]	58 (25.7)	24 (23.8)	34 (27.2)	0 (0)	0 (0)	0 (0)
Lapidus et al,[29] 2007	96*	49 (51.0)	47 (50.0)	Dalteparin 5000 units daily[a]	23[b]	37 (38.5)	18 (36.7)	19 (40.4)	0 (0)	0 (0)	0 (0)

Abbreviations: ATTP, antithrombotic pharmacologic prophylaxis; NA, not applicable; NS, not stated; UN, unknown.

* Total number of patients who underwent DVT surveillance.

[a] Both placebo and treatment groups received this dose for the first 7 postoperative days, placebo group then discontinued, treatment group continued for duration of immobilization.

[b] Mean duration of immobilization.

higher risk for development of DVT/PE and these patients received antithrombotic pharmacologic prophylaxis accordingly. The findings of the systematic review supports the findings that age greater than 40 years, obesity, cast immobilization, non–weight-bearing requirement, severe injury, and hindfoot surgery have a high predictive value for development of DVT/PE during conservative or postoperative management of foot and ankle disorders.

The weaknesses in our systematic review include the use of only 2 reviewers, restriction of the literature search to the English language, and the lack of consistent information in the studies included in the analysis. Although a systematic review is best performed with a minimum of 3 reviewers to avoid bias, the authors have performed several systematic reviews together and are well versed in the process of performing a systematic review.[37] Restriction of the literature search to the English language could have resulted in important publications being excluded. However, with the inclusion of only studies of clinical level of evidence I and II, it is doubtful that additional meaningful information would have altered the findings. The lack of consistent information in the included studies (ie, weight-bearing status, use of mechanical antithrombotic prophylaxis, and postoperative exercises) could have altered the incidence of DVT/PE; however, several studies did include enough information in this regard that the overall incidence of DVT/PE is unlikely to be much different than what was found.

SUMMARY

A systematic review of a wide range of electronic biomedical databases and references was undertaken to identify published material relating to the incidence of venous thromboembolism during conservative and postoperative management of foot and ankle disorders and the reduction of these events with the use of antithrombotic pharmacologic prophylaxis. Based on the inclusion criteria used, 8 publications (all level of clinical evidence I or II therapeutic studies) were included in the analysis, with 3 related to the conservative management of traumatic foot and ankle injuries and 5 related to the postoperative management of elective surgery and surgical repair of traumatic foot and ankle injuries.[22–36] The incidence of DVT/PE in both the conservative and postoperative management groups was low: 5.9% DVT and 0.03% PE, and 3.3% DVT and 0.12% PE, respectively. Incidence of DVT/PE in patients treated with any form of antithrombotic pharmacologic prophylaxis for any duration during the recovery period compared with those who received no antithrombotic pharmacologic prophylaxis was difficult to determine in relation to conservative management of disorders affecting the foot and ankle. However, more than half of the DVT reported in postoperative management of disorders affecting the foot and ankle, whether secondary to elective procedures performed or surgical repair of traumatic injury, occurred in patients who received no antithrombotic pharmacologic prophylaxis. The only 2 randomized, placebo-controlled, double-blinded studies included in the analysis involved postoperative management of traumatic injuries of the foot/ankle (ie, ankle fractures, Achilles tendon rupture repair) and found antithrombotic pharmacologic prophylaxis to significantly reduce the potential for development of DVT/PE, particularly after surgical repair of Achilles tendon rupture. The results of the included studies support the idea that cast immobilization, age greater than 40 years, non–weight-bearing requirement, obesity, severe injury and hindfoot surgery are all significant risk factors for the potential development of DVT/PE.

There is still little conclusive evidence for the protective effect of antithrombotic pharmacologic prophylaxis against development of DVT/PE during conservative and postoperative management of foot and ankle disorders. Given the devastating short-term and long-term mortality and morbidity of DVT/PE, the use of antithrombotic pharmacologic prophylaxis for foot and ankle disorders during conservative and post-operative management must be addressed with high-quality, prospective, random-ized, double-blinded, placebo-controlled studies with a minimum follow up of 60 days because of the combined mean time to diagnosis of DVT/PE from the pooled data of 35 days. Until that time, the decision to initiate, the type of antithrombotic phar-macological prophylaxis to use, and the duration of use following conservative or postoperative management of foot and ankle disorders should be based on known risk factors and a low threshold for DVT surveillance throughout healing.

REFERENCES

1. Batra S, Kurup H, Gul A, et al. Thromboprophylaxis following cast immobilization for lower limb injuries-survey of current practice in United Kingdom. Injury 2006; 37(9):813–81.
2. Biant LC, Hill G, Singh D. Antithrombotic prophylaxis in foot and ankle surgery in the UK. Presented at the British Orthopedic Foot and Ankle Society Annual Meeting, Cheshire, United Kingdom, 4–6 November 2004. Available at: http://www.bofas.org.uk/ProfessionalArea/PreviousMeetingsInformation/ArchiveofAbstracts/tabid/68/Default.aspx. Accessed on April 12, 2011.
3. Chen L, Soares D. Fatal pulmonary embolism following ankle fracture in a 17-year-old girl. J Bone Joint Surg Br 2006;88(3):400–1.
4. Clarke AM, Winson IG. Does plaster immobilization predispose to pulmonary embolism. Injury 1992;23(8):533–4.
5. Decramer A, Lowyck H, Demuynck M. Parameters influencing thromboprophy-laxis management of a lower leg trauma related with a cast/splint. Acta Orthop Belg 2008;74(5):672–7.
6. Gadgil A, Thomas RH. Current trends in thromboprophylaxis in surgery of the foot and ankle. Foot Ankle Int 2007;28(10):1069–73.
7. Hanslow SS, Grujie L, Slater HK, et al. Thromboembolic disease after foot and ankle surgery. Foot Ankle Int 2006;27(5):693–5.
8. Hatch DJ, Magnusson PG, DiGiovanni JE. Mini-dose heparin prophylaxis for high-risk patients in podiatric surgery. J Am Podiatry Assoc 1980;70(2):73–83.
9. Kroll HR, Odderson IR, Allen FH. Deep vein thrombi associated with the use of plastic ankle-foot orthosis. Arch Phys Med Rehabil 1998;79:576–8.
10. Lim W, Wu C. Balancing the risks and benefits of thromboprophylaxis in patients undergoing podiatric surgery. Chest 2009;135(4):888–90.
11. Nesheiwat F, Surgi AR. Deep venous thrombosis and pulmonary embolism following cast immobilization of the lower extremity. J Foot Ankle Surg 1996; 35(6):590–4.
12. Parsonage J. Venous thromboembolism in patients with below-knee plaster casts. Emerg Nurse 2009;16(10):32–5.
13. Slaybaugh RS, Beasley BD, Massa EG. Deep venous thrombosis risk assess-ment, incidence, and prophylaxis in foot and ankle surgery. Clin Podiatr Med Surg 2003;20:269–89.
14. Wang F, Wara G, Knoblich GO, et al. Pulmonary embolism following operative treatment of ankle fractures: a report of three cases and review of the literature. Foot Ankle Int 2002;23(5):406–10.
15. Wolf JM, DiGiovanni CW. A survey of orthopedic surgeons regarding DVT prophylaxis in foot and ankle trauma surgery. Orthopedics 2004;27(5):504–8.

16. Wukich DK, Waters DH. Thromboembolism following foot and ankle surgery: a case series and literature review. J Foot Ankle Surg 2008;47(3):243–9.
17. Geerts WH, Bergqvist D, Pineo GF, et al. Prevention of venous thromboembolism: American College of Chest Physicians Evidenced-Based Clinical Practice Guidelines (8th edition). Chest 2008;133:381s–453s.
18. Edmonds MJR, Crichten TJH, Runciman WB, et al. Evidence-based risk factors for postoperative deep vein thrombosis. ANZ J Surg 2004;74:1082–97.
19. Felcher AH, Mularski RA, Mosen DM, et al. Incidence and risk factors for venous thromboembolic disease in podiatric surgery. Chest 2009;135(4):917–22.
20. Kakkar VV, Howe CT, Nicolaides AN, et al. Deep vein thrombosis of the leg. Is there a "high-risk" group? Am J Surg 1970;120:527–30.
21. Schade VL, Roukis TS. Near fatal pulmonary embolus in a patient despite pharmacological and mechanical antithrombotic prophylaxis. a case report. Institutional Scientific Poster Presentation, American College of Foot and Ankle Surgeons 68th Annual Scientific Conference. Mandalay Bay, Las Vegas (NV), February 23–26, 2010.
22. Brown E, Bleotman A. Prophylaxis of venous thromboembolism in patients with lower limb plaster cast immobilization. Emerg Med J 2007;24(7):495–6.
23. Ettema HB, Kollen BJ, Verheyen CCPM, et al. Prevention of venous thromboembolism in patients with immobilization of the lower extremities: a meta-analysis of randomized controlled trials. J Thromb Haemost 2008;6(7):1093–8.
24. Jersmann HPA, Girard P, Murashige N, et al. Reviparin after leg injury requiring immobilization. N Engl J Med 2003;348(11):1061–3.
25. Jørgensen PS, Warming J, Hansen K, et al. Low molecular weight heparin (Innohep) as thromboprophylaxis in outpatients with a plaster cast a venographic controlled study. Thromb Res 2002;105:477–80.
26. Kock HJ, Schmit-Neuerburg KP, Hanke J, et al. Thromboprophylaxis with low-molecular-weight heparin in outpatients with plaster-cast immobilization of the leg. Lancet 1995;346:459–61.
27. Kujath P, Spannagel U, Habscheid W. Incidence and prophylaxis of deep venous thrombosis in outpatients with injury of the lower limb. Haemostasis 1993;23(Suppl 1):20–6.
28. Lapidus LJ, Poner S, Elvin A, et al. Prolonged thromboprophylaxis with Dalteparin during immobilization after ankle fracture surgery: a randomized placebo-controlled, double-blind study. Acta Orthop 2007;78(4):528–35.
29. Lapidus LJ, Rosfers S, Ponzer S, et al. Prolonged thromboprophylaxis with Dalteparin after surgical treatment of Achilles tendon rupture: a randomized, placebo-controlled study. J Orthop Trauma 2007;21(1):52–7.
30. Lassen MR, Borris LC, Nakov RL. Use of the low-molecular weight heparin reviparin to prevent deep-vein thrombosis after leg injury requiring immobilization. N Engl J Med 2002;347(10):726–30.
31. Mizel MS, Temple HT, Michelson JD, et al. Thromboembolism after foot and ankle surgery a multicenter study. Clin Orthop Relat Res 1998;348:180–5.
32. Patil S, Gandhi J, Cuzzon L, et al. Incidence of deep-vein thrombosis in patients with fractures of the ankle treated in a plaster cast. J Bone Joint Surg Br 2007;89(10):1340–3.
33. Radl R, Kastner N, Aigner C, et al. Venous thrombosis after hallux valgus surgery. J Bone Joint Surg Am 2003;85(7):1204–8.
34. Riou B, Rothman C, Lecoules N, et al. Incidence and risk factors for venous thromboembolism in patients with nonsurgical isolated lower limb injuries. Am J Emerg Med 2007;25:502–8.

35. Solis G, Saxby T. Incidence of DVT following surgery of the foot and ankle. Foot Ankle Int 2002;23(5):411–4.
36. Spannagel U, Kujath P. Low molecular weight heparin for the prevention of thromboembolism in outpatients immobilized by plaster cast. Semin Thromb Hemost 1993;19(Suppl 1):131–41.
37. Wright RW, Brand RA, Dunn W, et al. How to write a systematic review. Clin Orthop Relat Res 2007;455:23–9.
38. Kearon C. Natural history of venous thromboembolism. Circulation 2003;107: 122–30.
39. Lohr JM, Kerr TM, Lutter KS, et al. Lower extremity calf thrombosis: to treat or not to treat? J Vasc Surg 1991;14(5):618–23.
40. Micheli LJ. Thromboembolic complications of cast immobilization for injuries of the lower extremities. Clin Orthop Relat Res 1975;108:191–5.
41. Philbrick JT, Becer DM. Calf deep venous thrombosis. A wolf in sheep's clothing? Arch Intern Med 1988;148:2131–8.
42. Haas S. Deep vein thrombosis: beyond the operating table. Orthopedics 2000; 23(Suppl 6):s629–32.
43. Labropoulos N, Waggoner T, Sammis W, et al. The effect of venous thrombus location and extent on the development of post-thrombotic signs and symptoms. J Vasc Surg 2008;48(2):407–12.
44. Cirlincione AS, Mendicino R, Catanzariti AR, et al. Low-molecular-weight heparin for deep venous thrombosis prophylaxis in foot and ankle surgery: a review. J Foot Ankle Surg 2001;40(2):96–100.
45. Ponticello M, Steinberg J. Pertinent pointers on DVT prophylaxis. Podiatry Today 2007;20(4):83–90.
46. Wille-Jørgensen P, Jorgensen LN, Crawford M. Asymptomatic postoperative deep vein thrombosis and the development of postthrombotic syndrome. A systematic review and meta-analysis. Thromb Haemost 2005;93(2):236–41.
47. Leonardi MJ, McGory ML, Ko CY. The rate of bleeding complications after pharmacologic deep venous thrombosis prophylaxis. A systematic review of 33 randomized controlled trials. Arch Surg 2006;141:790–9.
48. Ward N, Ladher N, Sharp R. Compliance with self-administered deep vein thrombosis prophylaxis in foot and ankle patients. Presented at the British Orthopedic Foot and Ankle Society Annual Meeting. Cheshire (United Kingdom), November 4–6, 2009. Available at: http://www.bofas.org.uk/ProfessionalArea/Previous MeetingsInformation/ArchiveofAbstracts/tabid/68/Default.aspx. Accessed April 12, 2011.

Pigmented Villonodular Synovitis of the Distal Tibiofibular Joint: A Case Report

Andreas F. Mavrogenis, MD[a], Kleo T. Papaparaskeva, MD[b],
Spyros Galanakos, MD[a], Panayiotis J. Papagelopoulos, MD, DSc[a],*

KEYWORDS

- Pigmented villonodular synovitis • Distal tibiofibular joint
- Surgical treatment

Pigmented villonodular synovitis (PVNS) is a rare proliferative disorder of the synovium that affects young and middle-aged adults.[1–6] PVNS is usually monoarticular and often arises in the joints.[5] This condition may be locally destructive and involve muscles, tendons, bursae, bone, and skin.[6] The most common locations are the knee and hip, flexor tendon sheaths of the hand, ankle, and shoulder joints. The sternoclavicular and tibiofibular joints are rare locations.[7–10] Patients frequently present with pain, joint effusions, and swelling. The duration of symptoms varies.[5,11]

Plain radiographs may show defects in the adjacent bone, bone cysts, and a sclerotic rim.[12,13] Effusions may appear dense on plain radiographs and computed tomographic (CT) images because of high iron content. Magnetic resonance imaging (MRI) is useful to delineate the soft tissue extent and bone involvement, if present, of PVNS, showing low signal intensity on both T1- and T2-weighted images.[3,6] The extent of the abnormality may seem larger than it actually is because of the blooming phenomenon of the magnetic susceptibility effect caused by hemosiderin.[6,10] Macroscopically, PVNS appears as thickened reddish-brown synovium (because of hemosiderin deposition) with numerous villous projections. Microscopically, the lesions are composed of matted villi containing thin-walled vascular channels and supporting stroma closely packed with polyhedral stromal cells, multinucleate giant cells, and macrophages that

[a] First Department of Orthopaedics, Athens University Medical School, ATTIKON University Hospital, Rimini 1, Chaidari, 12462, Athens, Greece
[b] Department of Pathology, Athens University Medical School, ATTIKON University Hospital, Rimini 1, Chaidari, 12462, Athens, Greece
* Corresponding author.
E-mail address: pjportho@otenet.gr

Clin Podiatr Med Surg 28 (2011) 589–597
doi:10.1016/j.cpm.2011.04.005
0891-8422/11/$ – see front matter © 2011 Elsevier Inc. All rights reserved.

may contain hemosiderin and lipids. Abundant collagen, fibrosis, and hyalinization may be present in patients with long-standing PVNS.[1,2,6]

The incidence of PVNS in the ankle joint is approximately 2.5%,[11] but the occurrence in the distal tibiofibular joint is relatively rare.[14] This case report presents a patient with PVNS of the distal tibiofibular joint. To the best of the authors' knowledge, this case is only the second report in the English language medical literature of isolated involvement of the distal tibiofibular joint.

CASE REPORT

A 40-year-old man presented with a 3 months' history of edema of the left distal tibia and ankle (Fig. 1). His past medical history was unremarkable. The patient denied any previous trauma to the area. The results of the laboratory examinations were within normal values.

Radiographs of the left distal tibia and ankle joint showed irregularity of the distal tibiofibular joint (Fig. 2). The CT scan results showed erosion of the distal tibiofibular joint and a large soft tissue mass extending through both sides of the joint (Fig. 3). The MRI results showed a soft tissue mass with a maximal diameter of 95 mm, extending through the distal tibiofibular joint to the anterior and posterior compartments of the distal tibia with erosion of the tibia and fibula (Fig. 4). The bone scan results showed increased radioisotope uptake at the left distal tibia (Fig. 5). Histologic sections of the biopsy specimens showed proliferation of round to polygonal cells, with scant cytoplasm forming villous and fingerlike or rounded mass underlying the synovium. Multinucleated giant cells were scattered throughout the lesion. Hemosiderin-laden macrophages varied in number, giving the synovium a dark-brown appearance (Fig. 6). These findings were consistent with the diagnosis of PVNS.

Through the anterolateral (Fig. 7A) and posteromedial (see Fig. 7B) approaches, complete excision of the proliferative synovium was done (see Fig. 7C). Histologic evaluation of the excised specimen was consistent with the biopsy result. Postoperative recovery of the patient was uneventful. At the latest examination, 3 years after diagnosis and surgical treatment, MRI results showed no evidence of local recurrence (Fig. 8).

DISCUSSION

PVNS is a rare benign but locally destructive disease with significant potential for severe joint morbidity. This article presents a rare case of PVNS involving the distal tibiofibular joint.

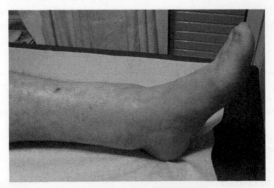

Fig. 1. Left leg and foot showing edema at the distal tibia.

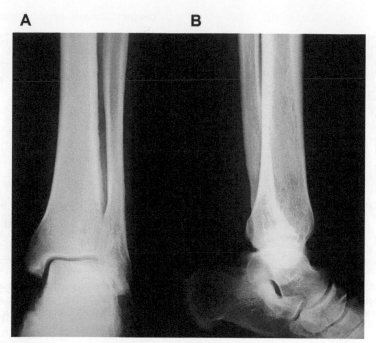

Fig. 2. (*A*) Anteroposterior and (*B*) lateral radiographs of the left distal tibia and ankle joint show irregularity of the distal tibiofibular joint.

The pathogenesis of PVNS remains uncertain. Trauma has been proposed to be the precipitating factor. Others have postulated that PVNS may be because of a chronic inflammatory process or a disorder of lipid metabolism.[2,15,16] However, some investigators have suggested that PVNS may be a neoplastic process because it may rarely

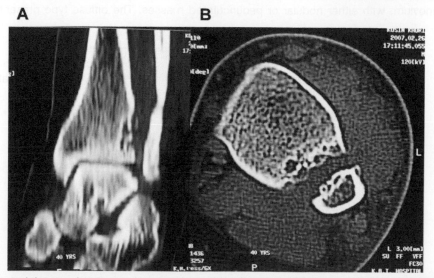

Fig. 3. (*A*) Coronal CT image shows erosion of the distal tibiofibular joint. (*B*) Axial CT image shows a large soft tissue mass extending through both sides of the joint.

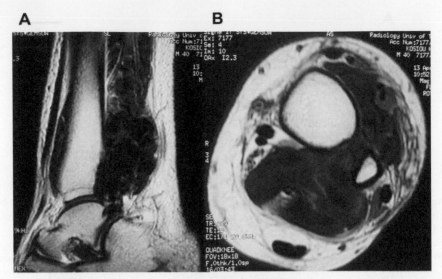

Fig. 4. (*A*) Sagittal and (*B*) axial magnetic resonance images show a soft tissue mass with a maximal diameter of 95 mm, extending through the distal tibiofibular joint to the anterior and posterior compartments of the distal tibia with erosion of the tibia and fibula.

metastasize and because there has been evidence that some lesions are monoclonal.[17–21] Granowitz and Mankin[22] classified PVNS into 3 types with similar histology, including villous synovial proliferation with microscopic villi, histiocytes, foam cells, and multinucleated giant cells. The isolated discrete type occurs within a tendon sheath, most often in the hand; this type has been termed giant cell tumor of the tendon sheath (GCTTS) and is currently genetically considered to be a separate entity from PVNS. The localized type occurs most commonly in the knee and usually presents with mechanical symptoms; it is characterized by focal involvement of the synovium, with either nodular or pedunculated masses. The diffuse type presents

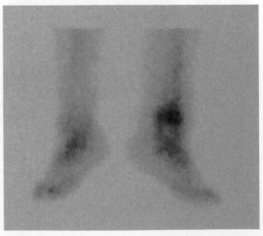

Fig. 5. Technetium Tc 99m bone scan image shows increased radioisotope uptake in the left distal tibia.

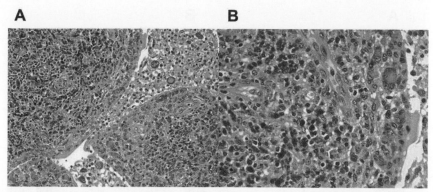

Fig. 6. (A) Proliferation of round to polygonal cells, with scant cytoplasm forming villous fingerlike or rounded mass underlying the synovium (hematoxylin-eosin, original magnification ×200). (B) Multinucleated giant cells are scattered throughout the lesion. Hemosiderin-laden macrophages vary in number, giving the synovium a dark-brown appearance (hematoxylin-eosin, original magnification ×400).

with chronic edema and pain, most commonly in the knee, hip, and ankle; it affects virtually the entire synovium.[22] The tenosynovial form is more common in the phalangeal region, metatarsal area, and retromalleolar groove, whereas the articular form is more common in the hindfoot and ankle. In the foot and ankle, the localized extra-articular form is more common than the diffuse intra-articular form. A more aggressive diffuse extra-articular form has also been described in the foot at a much higher rate than the traditional form.[23] Occasionally, a solitary intra-articular nodule (termed localized intra-articular PVNS or localized nodular synovitis) may occur.[24,25]

A combination of clinical, radiological, and histologic correlation is necessary for the diagnosis of PVNS. Plain radiographs alone are not confirmatory of this diagnosis despite the proper clinical presentation. Only 33% and 25% of the patients with diffuse and localized disease, respectively, manifested radiographic cysts or erosions secondary to osseous involvement.[10,12,26] In addition, the patients with radiographic

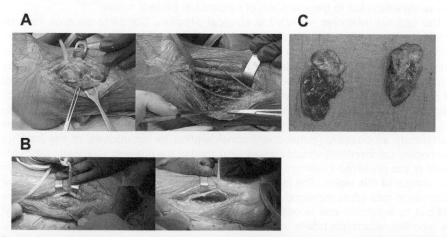

Fig. 7. Through the (A) anterolateral and (B) posteromedial approaches, (C) complete excision of the proliferative synovium was performed.

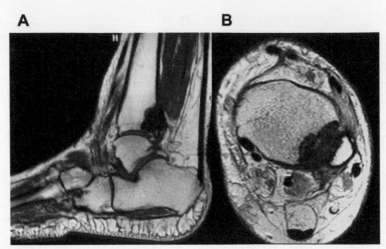

Fig. 8. At the latest examination, 3 years after diagnosis and surgical treatment, (*A*) sagittal and (*B*) axial magnetic resonance images show no evidence of local recurrence.

changes were those with more extensive disease involving bone. Of the patients with GCTTS, 15% can have erosive bony lesions, whereas among those with PVNS of the ankle, bone erosions are present in as much as 56% of cases.[27,28] Clinical correlation in these cases is used to differentiate between these different pathologic disease processes. MRI is a useful noninvasive means of diagnosis based on the unique, diffuse, hypodense infiltrative lesion involving soft tissue structures on T1- and T2-weighted images.[26,29–31] Findings on MRI are likely attributable to the hemosiderin deposition in the affected tissues. Hemosiderin causes a decrease in signal on both T1- and T2-weighted images. Although MRI is very sensitive in diagnosing these lesions, PVNS is nonspecific and is often confused with rheumatoid arthritis or soft tissue sarcoma. Recurrent GCTTS can also mimic soft tissue sarcoma clinically and on imaging studies. The radiologists reported 2 cases in the authors' series that were likely soft tissue sarcoma. The presence of erosive changes and extensive soft tissue extension led to the suspicion of sarcoma in these 2 cases.[29–31]

The optimal treatment of PVNS is surgical excision. Complete excision may be limited by the vicinity of the neurovascular bundle. In patients with localized disease, wide excision usually minimizes the chances of local recurrence, but recurrence may ensue if excision is inadequate. In patients with diffuse disease, total synovectomy has a much lower recurrence rate than partial synovectomy and is the preferred treatment of choice.[32] To ensure complete excision of the mass and the affected surrounding tissues, an open procedure should be performed on both sides of the joint for resection of abnormal tissues. Pathologic synovial tissues should be removed as completely as possible. Subsequent consideration for arthrodesis of the joint for secondary osteoarthritis should be well explained to the patients. Complete synovectomy is the preferred treatment of PVNS. Incomplete removal most likely results in recurrence of this lesion. The localized PVNS has an excellent prognosis and a low recurrence rate when managed surgically. The more common diffuse PVNS is more difficult to eradicate and is optimally treated with near-total or total synovectomy; its reported recurrence rate is up to 46%.[33]

Moderate-dose external beam radiation therapy may improve the likelihood of local control for patients with refractory cases and incompletely resected and unresectable

PVNS.[4,10,34–39] Adjuvant therapy with intra-articular instillation of radioactive isotopes (ie, dysprosium 165 or yttrium 90) or cryosurgical surface spray may be considered for patients thought to be at high risk for recurrence.[6,10,36,40–42]

REFERENCES

1. Jaffe HL, Lichtenstein L, Sutro CJ. Pigmented villonodular synovitis, bursitis and tenosynovitis. Arch Pathol 1941;31:731–65.
2. Granowitz SP, D'Antonio J, Mankin HL. The pathogenesis and long-term end results of pigmented villonodular synovitis. Clin Orthop Relat Res 1976;(114):335–51.
3. Mandelbaum BR, Grant TT, Hartzman S, et al. The use of MRI to assist in diagnosis of pigmented villonodular synovitis of the knee joint. Clin Orthop Relat Res 1988;(231):135–9.
4. Blanco CE, Leon HO, Guthrie TB. Combined partial arthroscopic synovectomy and radiation therapy for diffuse pigmented villonodular synovitis of the knee. Arthroscopy 2001;17:527–31.
5. Durr HR, Stabler A, Maier M, et al. Pigmented villonodular synovitis. Review of 20 cases. J Rheumatol 2001;28:1620–30.
6. Shabat S, Kollender Y, Merimsky O, et al. The use of surgery and yttrium 90 in the management of extensive and diffuse pigmented villonodular synovitis of large joints. Rheumatology (Oxford) 2002;41:1113–8.
7. Miller WE. Villonodular synovitis: pigmented and nonpigmented variations. South Med J 1982;75:1084–6, 1092.
8. González Della Valle A, Piccaluga F, Potter HG, et al. Pigmented villonodular synovitis of the hip: 2- to 23-year follow-up study. Clin Orthop Relat Res 2001;388:187–99.
9. Ryan RS, Louis L, O'Connell JX, et al. Pigmented villonodular synovitis of the proximal tibiofibular joint. Australas Radiol 2004;48(4):520–2.
10. Tyler WK, Vidal AF, Williams RJ, et al. Pigmented villonodular synovitis. J Am Acad Orthop Surg 2006;14:376–85.
11. Rao AS, Vigorita VJ. Pigmented villonodular synovitis (giant-cell tumor of the tendon sheath and synovial membrane). A review of eighty-one cases. J Bone Joint Surg Am 1984;66:76–94.
12. Bravo SM, Winalski CS, Weissman BN. Pigmented villonodular synovitis. Radiol Clin North Am 1996;34:311–26.
13. Valer A, Ramirez G, Massons J, et al. Pigmented villonodular synovitis of the wrist. Apropos of a case. Rev Chir Orthop Reparatrice Appar Mot 1997;83:164–7.
14. Mori H, Nabeshima Y, Mitani M, et al. Diffuse pigmented villonodular synovitis of the ankle with severe bony destruction: treatment of a case by surgical excision with limited arthrodesis. Am J Orthop (Belle Mead NJ) 2009;38(12):E187–9.
15. Flandry F, Norwood LA. Pigmented villonodular synovitis of the shoulder. Orthopedics 1989;12:715–8.
16. Sakkers RJ, de Jong D, van der Heul RO. X-chromosome inactivation in patients who have pigmented villonodular synovitis. J Bone Joint Surg Am 1991;73:1532–6.
17. Ray RA, Morton CC, Lipinski KK, et al. Cytogenetic evidence of clonality in a case of pigmented villonodular synovitis. Cancer 1991;67:121–5.
18. Fletcher JA, Henkle C, Atkins L, et al. Trisomy 5 and trisomy 7 are nonrandom aberrations in pigmented villonodular synovitis: confirmation of trisomy 7 in uncultured cells. Genes Chromosomes Cancer 1992;4:264–6.

19. Choong PF, Willen H, Nilbert M, et al. Pigmented villonodular synovitis. Monoclonality and metastasis—a case for neoplastic origin? Acta Orthop Scand 1995;66: 64–8.
20. Ohjimi Y, Iwasaki H, Ishiguro M, et al. Short arm of chromosome 1 aberration recurrently found in pigmented villonodular synovitis. Cancer Genet Cytogenet 1996;90:80–5.
21. Huracek J, Troeger H, Menghiardi B, et al. Malignant course of pigmented villonodular synovitis of the flexor tendon sheath of the small finger—case report and review of the literature. Handchir Mikrochir Plast Chir 2000;32:283–90.
22. Granowitz SP, Mankin HJ. Localized pigmented villonodular synovitis of the knee. Report of five cases. J Bone Joint Surg Am 1967;49:122–8.
23. Somerhausen NS, Fletcher CD. Diffuse-type giant cell tumor: clinicopathologic and immunohistochemical analysis of 50 cases with extraarticular disease. Am J Surg Pathol 2000;24:479–92.
24. Jelinek JS, Kransdorf MJ, Shmookler BM, et al. Giant cell tumor of tendon sheath: MR imaging findings in nine cases. Am J Roentgenol 1994;162:919–22.
25. Sharma H, Jane MJ, Reid R. Pigmented villonodular synovitis of the foot and ankle: forty years of experience from the Scottish bone tumor registry. J Foot Ankle Surg 2006;45(5):329–36.
26. Harris O, Ritchie DA, Maginnis R, et al. MRI of giant cell tumor of tendon sheath and nodular synovitis of the foot and ankle. Foot 2003;13:19–29.
27. Dorwart RH, Genant HK, Johnston WH, et al. Pigmented villonodular synovitis of synovial joints: clinical, pathologic, and radiologic features. Am J Roentgenol 1984;143:877–85.
28. Ushijima M, Hashimoto H, Tsunoyoshi M, et al. Giant cell tumor of the tendon sheath (nodular tenosynovitis). A study of 207 cases to compare the large joint group with the common digit group. Cancer 1986;57:875–84.
29. Llauger J, Palmer J, Monill JM, et al. MR imaging of benign soft-tissue masses of the foot and ankle. Radiographics 1998;18:1481–98.
30. Iovane A, Midiri M, Bartolotta TV, et al. Pigmented villonodular synovitis of the foot: MR findings. Radiol Med (Torino) 2003;106:66–73.
31. Cheng XG, You YH, Liu W, et al. MRI features of pigmented villonodular synovitis (PVNS). Clin Rheumatol 2004;23:31–4.
32. Ogilvie-Harris DJ, McLean J, Zarnett ME. Pigmented villo-nodular synovitis of the knee. The results of total arthroscopic synovectomy, partial, arthroscopic synovectomy, and arthroscopic local excision. J Bone Joint Surg Am 1992;74:119–23.
33. Flandry F, Hughston JC. Pigmented villonodular synovitis. J Bone Joint Surg Am 1987;69:942–9.
34. O'Sullivan TJ, Alport EC, Whiston HG. Pigmented villonodular synovitis of the temporomandibular joint. J Otolaryngol 1984;13:123–6.
35. O'Sullivan B, Cummings B, Catton C, et al. Outcome following radiation treatment for high-risk pigmented villonodular synovitis. Int J Radiat Oncol Biol Phys 1995; 32:777–86.
36. Chin KR, Barr SJ, Winalski C, et al. Treatment of advanced primary and recurrent diffuse pigmented villonodular synovitis of the knee. J Bone Joint Surg Am 2002; 84:2192–202.
37. Bisbinas I, De Silva U, Grimer RJ. Pigmented villonodular synovitis of the foot and ankle: a 12-year experience from a tertiary orthopedic Oncology Unit. J Foot Ankle Surg 2004;43:407–11.
38. Brien EW, Sacoman DM, Mirra JM. Pigmented villonodular synovitis of the foot and ankle. Foot Ankle Int 2004;25:908–13.

39. O'Sullivan B, Griffin A, Wunder J, et al. Sustained remission following radiation treatment for high-risk pigmented villonodular synovitis [abstract]. Int J Radiat Oncol Biol Phys 2005;63:S50.
40. Kat S, Kutz R, Elbracht T, et al. Radiosynovectomy in pigmented villonodular synovitis. Nuklearmedizin 2000;39:209–13.
41. Mohler DG, Kessler BD. Open synovectomy with cryosurgical adjuvant for treatment of diffuse pigmented villonodular synovitis of the knee. Bull Hosp Jt Dis 2000;59:99–105.
42. Mendenhall WM, Mendenhall CM, Reith JD, et al. Pigmented villonodular synovitis. Am J Clin Oncol 2006;29:548–50.

Index

Note: Page numbers of article titles are in **boldface** type.

A

Ablative arthroscopy, 454–455
Abraders, 442
Accessory anterior portal, 450
Achilles tendoscopy, 568
Anesthetics, 445
    for diagnostic injections, 461, 463–464
    for insufflation, 451
Ankle arthroscopy
    for anterior impingement, **491–510**
    for arthrodesis, **511–521**
    for fractures, 455, **523–538**
    for osteochondral lesions, 459–462, **481–490**
    for soft tissue pathology, **469–480**
    for trauma, 455, 482–483, **523–538**
    practical aspects of, **441–452**
    preoperative evaluation for, **453–467**
"Ankle impingement sign," 497
Ankle tendoscopy, **561–570**
    Achilles tendon, 568
    anatomic considerations in, 562
    contraindications for, 562–563
    flexor hallucis tendon, 568
    indications for, 562–563
    peroneal tendon, 566–567
    posterior tibial tendon, 567–568
    technique for, 563–565
    versus open treatment, 561
Anterior ankle impingement, **491–510**
    anterolateral, 491–494
    arthroscopic treatment of, 501–507
    causes of, 494–497
    clinical presentation of, 497–498
    conservative treatment of, 501
    distal fascicle of anterior inferior tibiofibular ligament and, 493–494
    imaging of, 498–501
    meniscoid lesion in, 492
    osteophytes in, 495–497
    synovitis in, 492
Anterocentral portal, 450
Anterolateral impingement test, 456

Clin Podiatr Med Surg 28 (2011) 599–605
doi:10.1016/S0891-8422(11)00060-7
0891-8422/11/$ – see front matter © 2011 Elsevier Inc. All rights reserved.
podiatric.theclinics.com

Anterolateral portal, 450
Anteromedial portal, 450
Antithrombotic therapy, **571–588**
    in conservative treatment, 575, 577–578
    in postoperative management, 576, 578–582, 584–585
"Around-the-world" approach, to examination, 456
Arthrodesis, arthroscopic, **511–521**
    contraindications for, 511–512
    indications for, 511–512
    outcomes of, 514–518
    subtalar joint, 548–549
    technique for, 512–513
Arthroereisis implants, removal of, 545–546
Arthroscopy
    anatomic considerations in, 448–450
    anesthesia for, 445
    contraindications to, 453–454
    for ankle arthrodesis, **511–521**
    for ankle injuries, **523–538**
    for anterior ankle impingement, **491–510**
    for osteochondral lesions, **481–490**
    for small joints, **551–560**
    for soft tissue pathology, 457–458, **469–480**
    hemostasis in, 445–446
    indications for, 453–455
    instrumentation for, 441–444, 540–541, 563–565
    insufflation in, 450–451
    joint distraction for, 446–448
    positioning for, 444
    practical aspects of, **441–452**
    preoperative evaluation for, **453–467**
    subtalar joint, **539–550**

B

Bandaging, for distraction, 447
Bassett lesions, 472–473
Bassett's ligament, 472–473, 493–494
Bony impingement, imaging of, 456–457
Bupivacaine, for diagnostic injections, 463–464
Burrs, 442

C

Calcaneal fractures, 546, 548
Calcium pyrophosphate dihydrate crystal deposition, 476–477
Capsular reflection, 449–450
Chondral-separated lesions, 482
Chondromatosis, synovial, 475–476
Computed tomography, 457–462

for anterior ankle impingement, 501
for osteochondral lesions, 484–485
for Wolin lesion, 472
Congenital disorders, soft tissue pathology in, 478
Conservative treatment, antithrombotic therapy for, 575, 577–578
"Crossover exam," 456
Crystalline deposition, 476–477
Curettes, 442
Cutters, 442
Cysts, osteochondral, 482–483

D

Debridement, of subtalar joint, 546
Deep venous thrombosis, prevention of. *See* Antithrombotic therapy.
Distal fascicle of anterior inferior tibiofibular ligament, anterior ankle impingement and,
    493–494
Dorsolateral portal, 450
Dorsomedial portal, 450

E

Epinephrine, for hemostasis, 445–446

F

Ferkel classification, of osteochondral lesions, 485
Fibrocartilaginous tissue, in Wolin lesion, 471–472
Fibular fractures, 533
Flexor hallucis tendoscopy, 568
Foot arthroscopy, **551–560**
    advantages of, 557
    anatomy of, 552–553
    complications of, 557–558
    diagnosis for, 554
    history of, 551–552
    indications for, 554–555
    physical examination for, 553–554
    planning for, 555
    technique for, 555–557
Fractures, **523–538**
    arthroscopically assisted treatment of
        assessment for, 524
        contraindications for, 524
        indications for, 523–524
        pearls in, 524–525
        pediatric, 525–526
        technique for, 525–537
    reduction of, 455
    subtalar joint, 546, 548
    types of, 523–524

G

Gouges, 442
Gout, 476–477
Graspers, 442

H

Hand instruments, 442
Hemosiderin deposits, in pigmented villonodular synovitis, 474–475
Heparin and derivatives, for conservative treatment and postoperative management, 571–588

I

Impingement, 470–471
    anterior, **491–510**
    bony, imaging of, 456–457
Injections, diagnostic, 461, 463–464
Instrumentation
    for ankle arthroscopy, 441–444
    for subtalar joint arthroscopy, 540–541
    for tendoscopy, 563–565
Interosseus ligament, repair of, 544–545
Intra-articular space, 449–450

J

Joint distraction, 446–448

K

Knives, 442

L

Lactated Ringer solution, for insufflation, 451
Laser thermoablative system, 442–443
Lateral central portal, 450
Loose bodies, imaging of, 456–457

M

Magnetic resonance imaging
    for anterior ankle impingement, 498–499
    for osteochondral lesions, 484–485
    for pigmented villonodular synovitis, 594
    for Wolin lesion, 472
Magnetic resonance imaging arthrography
    for anterior ankle impingement, 500–501
    for soft tissue pathology, 457–461

Maisonneuve fractures, 533
Malleolar fractures, 526–533
Medial midline portal, 450
Meniscoid lesion, in anterior ankle impingement, 492
Metatarsophalangeal joint, first, arthroscopy of, **551–560**
    advantages of, 557
    anatomy of, 552–553
    complications of, 557–558
    diagnosis for, 554
    history of, 551–552
    indications for, 554–555
    physical examination for, 553–554
    planning for, 555
    technique for, 555–557
Middle facet, resection of, 544
Milgram classification, of synovial chondromatosis, 475–476

N

Nerve block, for subtalar joint evaluation, 539
Nerve injury, in osteochondral lesion repair, 489
Nonunion, in arthrodesis, 516

O

Os trigonum, resection of, 544
Osteoarthritis, arthrodesis for, 511–512
Osteochondral lesions, **481–490**
    arthroscopic treatment of, 485–489
    diagnosis of, 484–485
    imaging of, 459–462
    pathophysiology of, 482–486
Osteophytes, in anterior ankle impingement, 495–497
Osteotomes, 442

P

Palpation tests, 456
Pediatric patients, fractures in, 525–526
Peroneal nerve injury, in anterior ankle impingement treatment, 507
Peroneal tendoscopy, 566–567
Pigmented villonodular synovitis, 474–475, **589–597**
Pilon fractures, 533
Plica syndrome, 478
Portals, 448–449
Posterolateral portal, 450
Posteromedial portal, 450
Postoperative management, antithrombotic therapy for, 576, 578–582, 584–585
Power instruments, 442
Preoperative evaluation, **453–467**

Preoperative (*continued*)
    arthroscopic categories for, 435–455
    history in, 455
    physical examination in, 456
Probes, 442
Pseudogout, 476–477
Punches, 442

R

Radiation therapy, for pigmented villonodular synovitis, 594–595
Radiofrequency rods, 442–444
Radiography
    for anterior ankle impingement, 498
    for bony impingement, 456–457
    for osteochondral lesions, 459–460, 484
Ray and Kriz classification, of anterior inferior tibiofibular ligament variations, 494
Reparative arthroscopy, 454
Rheumatic disease, soft tissue pathology in, 473–477
Rheumatoid arthritis, 477
Rods, magnetized, 442
Ronguers, 442

S

Saline solution, for insufflation, 451
Screw fixation, for arthrodesis, 513
Shavers, 442
Sinus tarsi syndrome, 543–544
Soft tissue pathology, **469–480**
    congenital, 478
    evaluation of, 457–458
    rheumatic, 473–477
    traumatic, 469–473
Split Achilles tendon portal, 450
Sprains
    in anterolateral impingement, 491–494
    soft tissue pathology in, 469–473
"Squeeze test," 456
Stirrup, for distraction, 447
Subchondral cysts, 483–484
Subtalar joint arthroscopy, **539–550**
    diagnostic tests for, 539–540
    instrumentation for, 540–541
    pathologic conditions suitable for, 543–549
    procedure for, 541–543
    results of, 540
    versus conservative treatment, 540
Survey, arthroscopic, 454
Synovial chondromatosis, 475–476
"Synovial shelves," in anterior ankle impingement, 492
Synovitis, 470

in anterior ankle impingement, 492
pigmented villonodular, 474–475, 589–597

T

Talar fractures, 533–537
Tarsometatarsal joint, arthroscopy of, 558
Tendoscopy, ankle, **561–570**
Tenosynovectomy, for rheumatoid arthritis, 477
Thermoablative tools, 442–444
Thrombosis, prevention of. *See* Antithrombotic therapy.
Tibial tendon, tendoscopy of, 567–568
Tibiofibular joint, pigmented villonodular synovitis of, **589–597**
Tibiofibular ligament, accessory anterior inferior, 472–473, 493–494
Tillaux fractures, 525–526
Tourniquet, for hemostasis, 445–446
Trauma
    fractures, 455, **523–538**
    osteochondral lesions from, 482–483
    soft tissue, 469–473
Triplane fractures, 525–526

W

Weights, for distraction, 447
Wolin lesions, 471–472

Printed and bound by CPI Group (UK) Ltd, Croydon, CR0 4YY

03/10/2024

01040459-0016